End Insomnia
and Sleeping Problems
Without Drugs

ROSANNA D'AGNILLO

ISBN: 978-1484958292
ISBN-13: 1484958292

DEDICATION

For Zio Mario Del Papa.

I understood where your mind had gone and why, and wish I could have helped you.

CONTENTS

ACKNOWLEDGMENTS

Thank you to my guides for helping me survive the insomnia abyss and for helping me complete this book. Thanks to my children for being so beautiful, perfect as you are, and for making all the simple things in life so magical and memorable. Thanks to my husband Nikolai for his quiet support during the months I spent writing this book.

ROSANNA D'AGNILLO

"The most difficult battles in life are those
we fight within the mind."
--Chinese proverb

ROSANNA D'AGNILLO

INTRODUCTION

Welcome to my story of insomnia and sleeping problems and how I fixed them by myself, without drugs and without doctors. I'm not a doctor. I'm not a psychologist. I'm not an expert on sleep problems, except my own. I experienced difficulty sleeping for about ten years, and then severe insomnia for five years after this, from the years 2005 to 2010.

In fact, I've been awake most of the night for a long time. Since my mid-twenties.

I'd like to say I spent much of this time trying to figure out how to help myself, and that this book is the result of those thousands of hours of painstaking research, of trial and error as I self-experimented.

Actually, I spent most of this time really angry that I couldn't sleep. Mostly I fumed in black rage. After I figured out how to help myself, and after I made the commitment to restore my sleep health, the healing happened a lot more quickly than it took me to get down into the insomnia abyss in the first place.

It was a journey through total despair and—thank goodness—eventual success. I feel like Orpheus who escaped the underworld alive. I really feel like I've been to the other side and back. I'm scarred from the experience, as was he, but *I* made it and so can you.

You are not alone. You are not crazy. Getting a good night's sleep is not asking too much of life. Getting a good night's sleep is what you need in order to enjoy living.

I feel lucky and grateful to have even survived severe long-term insomnia. I know some people who have not survived, and it is to those that I dedicate this book.

I am now able to sleep between five to seven hours in a row. For insomniacs, this is an incredible amount of sleep. It's a light-year of sleep. Sleeping aids did not help me sleep. I consulted with numerous traditional medical professionals and not one was able to help me. I only received prescriptions for sleeping pills, anti-depression pills and recommendations for minor habit and environmental changes, like a bath before bed and no television in the bedroom.

Once I was on the path that made sense for me, it took about a year to teach myself to sleep again. Now when I wake up in the middle of the night, I'm usually able to fall back asleep. I can even get up and go to the bathroom and usually fall back asleep.

Does all of this make you flame with jealousy and longing? Read on, *padawan*, and I will share my tale with you. This book is not only for severe insomniacs. Anyone with sleeping problems will benefit from these strategies. It's not only your sleep that will benefit either. The positive changes cascade to the rest of your life, because of the way our minds and bodies are so interconnected, and because of the importance of sleep to every aspect of healthy and optimal functioning.

During my decade and a half of sleeping problems and since, I have met many people whose lives, health and families were destroyed or are in the process of being destroyed by sleep deprivation. Very serious depression and health problems. Divorce. Lost jobs. Abandoned passions. Truant children. And more. Even suicide. It's real and it's bad. Sleeplessness is not just a problem for those who are sleepless, but for their families, too. The impact cascades to their friends, their workplaces—and thus it billows out to our society as a whole.

In 2006, when I tried to speak with friends or family about my sleeping crisis, most would just ask me, kind of blankly, "Well, why don't you just roll over and go back to sleep?"

No, they were not joking. They simply could not understand just why the simple task of sleeping was so hard for me. Not funny for me at all. I had no one to talk to. No one who understood what I was going through. The isolation and a sense of my own misfit weirdness, my defective hardware, compounded the problem.

A lot has changed in the last few years. Today, I count many people even in my own small circle of family, friends and colleagues who have serious problems sleeping. Now, at the time of writing this book, nearly every woman over forty that I know has trouble sleeping at night! Both of my parents, my sister and my brother have problems sleeping. All of my aunts have problems sleeping. Impossible as this was to believe a few years ago, I am now one of the most well-rested people I know.

There is also increased media attention to the growing problem of sleep deprivation. My local newspaper features a weekly article about how to improve your sleep. I see more headlines on Yahoo about sleep deprivation than even a couple years ago. Many studies cited in the media stress the importance of sleep to our health, to our jobs, to our happiness, and to our children. In March 2013, the U.S. Centers for Disease Control and Prevention declared insufficient sleep to be a public health epidemic. Recent studies delineate the clear link between sleep deprivation and impaired performance in many disciplines and areas, from school-aged children to veterans to professional athletes.

Most of the popular environment and habit suggestions for improving your sleep are of limited value, especially for those who suffer from severe insomnia. Lavender, a warm bath before bed and cutting out the afternoon Starbucks have basically zero impact on severe insomnia.

What is severe insomnia? I spent five years sleeping less than three hours per day. Often I did not sleep these three hours in a row; I'd catch thirty minutes here and an hour there. At my worst I was sleeping just an hour or two every third day.

Sometimes when I tell people about this now, they don't believe me. They don't believe your body can survive on such little sleep. But it can, just not very well. They don't believe you can stay awake for so long without sleep. You can, but you sure feel crazy and really terrible.

I know it happened. Why? Because I was awake the whole time, counting—the seconds, the minutes, the hours—night after night, year after year, watching the clock.

As you can imagine, in this condition of severe insomnia, you are pretty messed up. The physical and mental consequences are terrible and life-changing.

It is for this reason that I feel compelled to add my voice to the discussion about sleeping problems.

My ideas are not pharmaceutical or quick-fixes. There are no pharmaceutical answers or quick fixes. If you're holding out for a special pill, you're out of luck.

You need to teach yourself how to sleep again. So-called sleeping pills only make it harder. As stupid as it seems, sleeping pills actually prevent you from reaching deep sleep. And they create a new host of problems that are far worse than your original insomnia.

You will need to commit some time and thought to your own process. I know this seems hard when you're so exhausted from sleeping poorly, but the rewards of your self-discovery are numerous, immediate and they are long-term. You will be a better person and live a more fulfilling, happy life because of your efforts.

You are worth it! I wish you patience and hope along this journey out of the abyss!

1 INSOMNIA IS A MEDICAL EMERGENCY

There's a reason sleep deprivation is used as a method of torture. It works like this: the victims of sleep-deprivation torture are kept awake for days at a time, and each time they doze off they're awakened and questioned.

At one point in his life, Menachem Begin, the Israeli prime minister from 1977 to 1983, and Nobel Peace Prize winner in 1978, was a prisoner of the former Soviet Union's KGB. Below he describes his experience of sleep deprivation:

> In the head of the interrogated prisoner, a haze begins to form. His spirit is wearied to death, his legs are unsteady, and he has one sole desire: to sleep...Anyone who has experienced this desire knows that not even hunger and thirst are comparable with it. [1]

Sound familiar? Only when I read this quote was I able to gauge that I was in terrible condition. When people tell you that you're exaggerating, you can tell them about Mr. Begin's time with the good ole KGB.

This was me with my firstborn. My birthing experience was a good substitute for Soviet interrogators. I had planned for a peaceful natural birth. I'd prepared with self-hypnosis so I could go without an epidural. I showed up to the hospital after my water broke, enthusiastic, with my birthing ball under one arm and my birthing plan in the other hand. Two quarts of hot raspberry leaf uterine tea waited in my backpack thermos, along with my favorite Yo Yo Ma recordings and a handful of special crystals.

---

[1] From his autobiography White Nights: The Story of a Prisoner in Russia.

To my surprise, I rapidly developed HELLP syndrome when labor got rolling. This is a life-threatening complication that is considered a variant or complication of pre-eclampsia. In a nutshell, being in labor disagreed with me greatly. I had liver and kidney failure. I could not have survived a C-section due to a platelet problem, so I was given the maximum dose of Pitocin to speed up contractions and dilation. I started having seizures so I was pumped full of anti-seizure medications and kind of tied to the operating table. I had an IV in each arm and a catheter in my bladder. I could not move except for the seizing. Because of the strength of the Pitocin dosage, I endured terrible agony during contractions, but could not be given any painkillers since they would slow down labor.

This lasted for about thirty delightful hours. I lost 1.6 liters of blood (that's more than three pints). I had to stay in the hospital four more days, during which time I had blood drawn every two hours to determine how my major organs were faring. My arms were so bruised from the needles that attendants poked around the veins in my hands and wrists. I was black and blue from elbow to fingertips for several weeks afterward.

How I Lost the Ability to Sleep

In summary, I was awake for four days and nights in a hostile environment. As you can imagine, I was really stressed out and scared, for me and my baby. I had not slept well for years, and had not slept much at all during the last half of my pregnancy because of back pain and constant bathroom trips. I was already down to a few hours of sleep per night or less. By the time I had my son, I was chronically sleep deprived and deeply exhausted. During my hospital stay, every time I started to doze off someone would wake me up for more poking and prodding and to provide baby-related instruction, even in the middle of the night. Even when I begged the nurses, in tears, to leave me undisturbed until sunrise, they refused because of the tests required. Whatever anti-seizure drugs were in me were in my son too, so my baby was sick and crabby.

When I left the hospital I was a total wreck. I was told it would take my son a week or so to process the anti-seizure medication. He screamed a lot. As a first-time mom and a high-strung woman, I found this extremely stressful. Since I was so sick, my milk didn't come in for ten days. Stupidly, I was determined not to supplement him with formula for the first few days. He started peeing out crystals and screamed non-stop. My lovely son and I had a completely miserable beginning to our physical life together.

To top it off, he was a very poor sleeper, too! As a newborn he was up every twenty or thirty minutes, and this lasted until he was at least fifteen months old. He never had that sleepy newborn phase. Rigorously, I tried all the well-known methods to no avail. All the way across spectrum from "Baby Wise" hard core sleep training to the "No Cry" Solutions, to "Happiest Baby on the Block" and total attachment parenting. After 15 months, he slept a maximum of 2 hours at a time, and could scream two hours at a time in the middle of the night. My son was one of those few unfortunate kids who experience night terrors. It was really weird. He looked wide awake; he'd be lying or standing in his crib eyes wide open and screaming his guts out, but he was not awake, and I could not awaken him, nor help him, only watch and wait for him to collapse into a short fitful sleep. Then he'd start up again with the screaming, eyes wide open but fast asleep.

To watch your baby scream for hours at a time, not understanding the cause of his suffering and unable to alleviate it, is very stressful for a new mother. We lived in a small one-bedroom apartment with paper-thin walls in a big Californian city. Our neighbors resented the nighttime screaming. They complained repeatedly to the manager. This made me even more uncomfortable and agitated because we didn't have the money to move to a bigger and more private place.

The result of all this? During these months I completely lost the ability to sleep normally, even for an hour at a time. My husband and I took shifts, but while he was "on duty" I remained so agitated, just waiting for and dreading the next round of screaming, that I could not fall or stay sleep. If I fell asleep, it was for a few minutes at a time, and then I'd jerk wide awake with my heart pounding, ready to puke.

Insanely, I was also pumping breast-milk every two hours, sometimes every hour, until he was six months old. Since I was up anyway, why not pump? I knew that the more I pumped, the more milk I'd make, and I thought that if he'd eat enough, he'd stop crying. As it happens, he was an enormous baby and a voracious eater, drinking more than two quarts of breast milk per day before he was a month old—I know because I obsessively measured every cubic millimeter of my pumped milk. In retrospect I should have supplemented. Not because the milk wasn't enough, or not fatty—in fact he was a whopping twenty pounds by four months old, with more rolls than the Michelin man. But rather, perhaps my milk was full of my stress hormones, and that probably didn't do my son any good. As a new mom, I simply didn't know any better, and I was extremely nervous about doing the right thing. I found it impossible to relax. There was no knowledgeable woman to help me, and no one to tell me to chill out, and no one I felt I could impose on to help me out.

As a musician, I ran my own business and didn't have maternity pay to tide me over. If I was wasn't working, I didn't have enough money to pay for my living expenses. Instead of trying to teach myself to sleep, I would nurse, pump, compose a jingle, wait on tip-toe, doze; nurse, pump again, do a voiceover, doze—all night long. I did numerous hours of voiceovers before my son even turned one, all in the middle of the night.

I've read about how the British Ministry of Defense reset soldiers' body clocks so they could go without sleep for up to 36 hours. They did this by putting small optical fibers in special glasses worn by the soldiers. The fibers project a ring of bright white light with a spectrum identical to a sunrise around the edge of the soldiers' retinas, fooling them into thinking they had just woken up. Apparently this was first tried on American pilots during the bombing of Kosovo.

I needed something like this for me, to help me manage the ridiculous schedule of working and pumping at night, and caring for the baby all day. My rest was never a priority, never even a consideration. I just assumed that any day my baby would start sleeping, and then I would be sleeping, too. I wanted to be a "normal mom", and enjoy motherhood.

But truth was, I often hated it. It was a prison for me. My baby didn't sleep and so neither did I, ever. I grew increasingly full of despair when he was three months old, and lapsed into serious post-partum depression. I did my best to conceal it, since only a weak, ungrateful, unnatural mother could feel so terrible all the time. I now understand the post-partum depression was caused by the insomnia.

My eldest had just turned two when my second son was born, and by this time I was totally messed up, trying to care for another big, crabby, difficult newborn and a busy toddler with night terrors, all while trying to make a living as an independent musician. It was an impossible, untenable situation. I thought I was responsible for fixing it all, for managing motherhood and my business with a smile, and if I couldn't, then I was a failure. I didn't have any family help and I didn't have enough money to hire help.

8

The physical and mental toll of this extended period of chronic severe insomnia was traumatic. In fact, I now recognize that I experienced a prolonged medical emergency. When you are extremely sleep deprived for a long time, you are not lazy. You are not crazy, although you will become crazy if you don't solve your problem. You are not a failure. You are not too sensitive or too fussy. What you are is sick.

You are not crazy. Or lazy. Or a loser. You are sick.

My Chinese sign happens to be an ox, and this describes my stubborn character to a fault, so I pushed on despite the armada of symptoms signaling this medical emergency, hoping it would all just go away on its own. Imagine you were going to your annual check-up with your physician. Last year, you were pretty healthy, fit, energetic, and enthusiastic, even though you'd been having some problems sleeping. Now you have these concerns to share:

Physical problems

- Old bone breaks refracturing.
- Severe abdominal pain (which turned out to be a benign but grapefruit-sized tumor in my liver.)
- Numerous palpable growths in my thyroid mass.
- High blood pressure and very high resting heart rate (often about 100-120 bpm for me!)
- Heart palpitations.
- Major gum loss and tooth decay / cavities in *every* molar.
- Easy to bruise, with the bruises lasting months.
- Constant muscle and joint aches and strains that wouldn't go away and that are easily provoked into a crisis whereby I couldn't walk, sleep or sit comfortably for weeks at a time.
- Increased sensitivity to pain. I couldn't stand being touched, poked, tickled, or massaged.
- No sex drive. I mean, *zero*. I used to be a really busy sexual person, horny as a goat for as long as I can remember, but during my insomnia period I was basically dead from the neck down.
- Terrible upper and lower back pain. Ribs and vertebrae never aligned comfortably.

9

- Cuts that don't heal and develop into infections. Infected fingernails and hangnails.
- Sudden graying of hair.
- Rapid loss of vision, both near and far. Rapid eye fatigue. Difficulty focusing.
- Fainting spells.
- Numerous and huge sties in my eyes that wouldn't go away, even after a year. Constant itching and redness.
- Chronic cold sores.
- Chronic bladder infections and staph infections in the pharynx and larynx.
- Chronic nausea, indigestion and constipation.
- New sensitivity and allergies to many types of foods, like canola oil, soy sauce, and cheese.
- Extreme sensitivity to smell & nausea easily induced, for example, just by walking down the household products isle at a grocery store.
- Very painful migraines that last for several days at a time.
- Loss of balance and extreme vertigo while walking, resting, driving, working. My surroundings would be spinning around, just like when you're tipsy and have the spins. Merry-go-rounds and even preschooler carnival rides with my kids were totally out of the question; I had my own private axis around which I was constantly spinning. (Vertigo is most often due to a processing problem with the inner ear and eyes. The vestibulocochlear nerve sends signals from the ear to the brain about where we are located in space, and correlates this position with the input from your eyes. So when the information from these systems is distorted, vertigo results.)
- Increased sensitivity to light and sound to the point where being outside is unbearable.
- Rapid weight gain and insatiable appetite, especially for fatty foods like cheese and meat.
- Water retention and painful swelling in the ankles, to the point where it was hard to sit or drive for long.
- Extreme and constant fatigue: unable to do routine, low-demand tasks like climb the stairs or fold laundry without pausing to rest. Even basic self-care like getting dressed, taking a shower, or

putting on a seatbelt felt like a burdensome imposition. *Why is every single thing so hard?* I literally did not have the strength to lace up boots. I spent the unusually frigid Calgary winter of 2008 with wet, cold feet in Crocs. I didn't care; I simply could not bend over for the time it took to sort out the boots. I did not have the focus or dexterity to manage shoelaces. I'd be too dizzy to straighten up; maybe I'd faint. Or my back would be too sore to bend over and then I wouldn't be able to get up. When my second child was born, I think I went at least four weeks without washing my hair—it was just too much work; I simply could not lift my arms above my head for the time it took to scrub my scalp and rinse out the shampoo. That is how physically diminished I was.

- Unable to do my job proficiently. I lost about 4 whole tones from the top of my voice—that's a lot—and even more from the bottom. I could no longer remember or perform any difficult or long piece, either vocally or on the piano. Coloratura (fast & light) singing was out of the question. Vocal fatigue arrived after 10 minutes of easy repertoire. Coordinating voiceovers for prerecorded videos was very difficult; I didn't have the reflexes to match up my voice to the video. Songs I'd had memorized for twenty, even thirty years I was no longer able to remember, or even play when looking at the sheet music. It was as though my brain, eyeballs, and hands were no longer connected in a way that let me make music and do music recording.

- Unable to negotiate the normal physical demands of mothering, like being patient with very young children. Carrying them, disciplining them in public. Strapping them into their car seats. Changing and washing their clothes. Feeding and caring for them.

- Loss of physical reflexes for even routine tasks like catching a ball, playing sports, driving and riding a bike.

- Trembling hands & loss of fine motor skills. In addition to not being able to play the piano, I couldn't put in my contact lenses, apply make-up, color within the lines of a picture. Even when my hands were not trembling, they would jerk around.

- Sleep paralysis, where you think you're awake, you see lots of weird stuff that you are probably dreaming about, but you think is real, yet your body is still atonic (as in REM sleep) so you can't move.

- Sleep inertia, where upon wakening you have a strong urge to just get back asleep, for hours afterward.

Cognitive Problems

- Inability to correctly perceive audio and visual stimuli. For example, when driving in traffic, it appeared that all the cars were coming at me and going to hit me; I could no longer discern well enough to make lane changes or get through a four-way stop sign. I was no longer able drive safely at night: I couldn't stay in my lane. When walking up stairs, I had to hold the railing because it seemed the stairs were jumping up at me, and I couldn't tell where to put my feet. If I was out walking with my kids, I couldn't tell from which direction a loud noise originated and if it was a threat to us.

- Frequent slurred, unintelligible speech and constant switching of consonants and vowels in words and sentences. For example, "let's watch this show, boys" comes out as "wets latch this shoy, bows."

- Unable to remember the names of common household or grocery items, or the names of friends, without thinking hard. Unable to do even simple addition in my head. What is my zip code? Did she give me the right change?

- Other reduced verbal abilities: unable to find a word. Not the *mot just* or a *bon mot*, but merely any simple word. Pass me the, uh, cheese. That's it; that's what it's called. The cheese. Unable to speak my second languages with any comprehensibility, French and Italian. In fact, I now mix up French, Italian, Russian and Spanish quite seamlessly and absurdly. Unable to tell jokes or stories, remember a punch line, sequence a narrative, give directions, describe any issue in a comprehensible way. I'd given up opening my mouth in a public forum, because nothing of any intelligibility could emerge from that orifice.

- Short term memory loss to the point of creating danger and professional/personal problems. Crippling self-doubt accompanies this symptom: did I shut off the stove? Did I leave my wallet and the groceries in the store, again? What do you mean you leant me that gold necklace? I have absolutely no idea where that money is. I have no memory of our conversation or that agreement.

- Long term memory loss - the years between about eleven and thirty-five for me are mostly gone. I have some vague memories, but am often not able to recall a major event even when prompted, for example, if I emceed a wedding or performed at a certain festival, even when I see a photo. All the days and nights just blur together without distinction. As an opera singer and pianist I have literally hundreds of songs stashed in my brain that I've been playing and singing since I was a young child. During my insomniac period, I could only play and sing a handful of simple pieces from memory.

- Inability to make quick decisions on any simple topic: Which line should I get in? Which credit card do I use? What did I come here for?
- Inability to problem-solve and apply basic reasoning, eg: identify a goal, set up actions and deadlines, and gauge progress. Simple issues become insurmountable hurdles.

Psychological problems

- Inability to navigate the perfectly regular and simple stresses of life. Crowds; traffic; a long checkout line; a messy kitchen; family arguments; rebellious kids. These things seem completely overwhelming and induce shut-down and a catastrophic sense of despair.
- Irrational and severe paranoia, blind rage and anger that soured all my relationships. Constant victim thinking. Negative fantasies of improbable and dangerous situations. For example, I kept feeling that my children would get injured everywhere and anywhere, or that my family would be the victim of random violence, etc.
- Very suicidal. Relentless urge to kill yourself so you'll be free and everyone will be rid of your useless worthless self. Wishing my children had never been cursed to a life of misery with me, and a strong belief that we'd all be better off dead.
- Severe depression. Severe post-partum depression. No interest or pleasure in life. "The cup" doesn't appear even half-empty, but totally void, shattered and irreparable. Chronic thoughts of worthlessness and harsh self- judgment.
- No interest in anything. Not exercise, books, creative pursuits, new recipes, games, challenges, any novelty, friends, movies, vacations, hosting or attending a party. It's not about an inability to find pleasure in these things; the problem is that everything feels like a Herculean amount of work, and it's just not worth the effort.

- Enormous, uncontrollable mood swings. Some big "ups" and lots of Marianas-Trench "downs."

If you reported this list of symptoms to your doctor, what do you think s/he'd do? You guessed it. You might be sent to a hospital's urgent care. At the least you'd get in queue for a zillion tests.

Where do you think Mr. Begin went when he got out of the KGB holding cell? Not straight back to work, that's for sure. Yet that's what we insomniacs expect of ourselves.

You might recognize in yourself some of these well recognized effects of sleep deprivation:

- Irritability
- Cognitive impairment
- Memory lapses; loss of short term and long term memory
- Impaired moral judgment
- Severe yawning
- Hallucinations
- Symptoms similar to ADHD, eg, inability to focus on a task.
- Impaired immune system
- Risk of type 2 diabetes
- Increased heart rate variability
- Risk of heart disease
- Increased reaction time
- Decreased accuracy
- Tremors
- Aches
- Growth suppression
- Risk of obesity

Suicidal?

Sleep deprivation alone is serious business, let alone long term insomnia. You don't have to be suicidal for insomnia to wreak havoc on your personality, to diminish your professional and personal life, and to seriously impair your basic and fine motor skills. War veterans who have problems sleeping are at higher risk for suicidal thoughts, according to a recent study from the Durham VA Medical Center in North Carolina. In teens and young adults, increased suicidal thoughts are also associated with sleep deprivation.

That said, if you are suicidal, put this book down and call a hotline right now. Just do it. They are great. They can help you. They know what to say, and sometimes it's good to talk to a stranger. I called a post-partum support hotline. Ain't no shame in admitting it. It was my avenue to some really good help at a time when I had no one else to talk to, and felt there was no hope. At the time, my mind and body were so weakened from years of sleeplessness that I was incapable of reading, internalizing and acting upon a self-help book. In addition to calling a hotline, you can speak to someone close to you, your doctor, a spiritual guide or a counselor, right away.

If you are so screwed up from insomnia that you are no longer interested in or able to engage in self-help, you need external help right away. Describe your physical symptoms instead of judging yourself as depressed. You can tell your family, or doctor, or friends that you are experiencing chronic insomnia, you're extremely weak, and are no longer capable of self-directing your healing. Ask for help in making a plan. Ask them to read this book and help you carry out the actions.

Give Yourself Permission to Seek Help

I'm not saying you need to get admitted to a hospital. In fact, as I'll speak about later, from my own personal experience, I don't think the traditional medical and psychiatric systems in North America have much useful care to offer the insomniac. But, what you do need is help. You need to give yourself permission to seek help. Insomnia and sleeping problems do not usually go away on their own. To the contrary, things get worse, and sometimes very quickly. Don't wait until you're too far gone to ask for help! If you don't get help sooner, you might be too incapacitated to ask for it later.

When you're vomiting and your throat aches, and your temperature is very high, do you pretend everything is fine? No. You call in sick. You cancel that dinner party. You stop worrying about the laundry pile and the sticky floor and getting that workout in. You say, "I'm going to lie down." You know that if you don't rest, you won't heal, and you'll make others sick, too.

In other words, you give yourself permission take a break. You step out of your routine and you put your mind in the right gear to heal yourself. You hunker down and start solving your problem. You don't expect instant results. You just dedicate some time and space and money to your recovery. You place your intention to heal yourself out there in our thought-soup, and you take some meaningful action to support it. You know there is no choice: if you fight the flu, you only prolong it.

It is the same with your sleeping problem. Your problem is a medical emergency. Give yourself permission to ask for and receive help. Give yourself permission to take the necessary time and energy to complete the healing. Are you ready for that? I hope so, for your sake. If you are reading this book, your mind is already in gear. Well done. If you want to fix your sleeping problem, there is no alternative; you must set your trajectory and follow through with action.

Sleep is Our Most Powerful Medicine

We are holistic beings, connected in mind and body. Sleep is one of our most powerful medicines. From my own personal experience, sleep has the most significant impact on my mood, strength, energy and clarity—more than diet or the other self-care I practice. I'm a piggy, and I can get a way with a few days of over-eating and still function normally. I can miss a couple days of meditation and exercise and still feel fit and balanced. Not so with under-sleeping. If for some reason I get less than 4 hours sleep, I feel really awful, all day long. I'll continue to feel awful until I get my 5-7 hours. Until that happens, all my waking hours are basically a total write-off.

Sleep provides massive restoration on so many levels. Scientists still don't understand exactly what it does but are learning just how important it is to health, normal functioning and longevity. What's clear is that without sleep we cannot maintain even minimum health in mind or body. If you suffer from insomnia, you probably don't need another medical study to tell you just how important sleep is. It's pretty simple.

Without sleep you don't enjoy being alive.
Without sleep your body stops working.

If you don't want to go crazy and get deathly ill, as of this moment you have only one simple goal in life: restoring healthy sleep habits and patterns. Everything else you're doing needs to go on the backburner for now. Spending that extra hour with your husband after the kids go to bed? Nope. Catching your favorite show at 10 pm? No way. Getting that extra chapter polished in the middle of the night? Forget about it.

This doesn't mean you need to sacrifice or abandon your fun, or your ambitions and bigger life goals. In fact, with healthy sleep you can accomplish whatever you want a lot faster and have a lot more fun doing it. You will be a better person to live with, to work with, to play with. You will be easier to love, and you will give love more easily. In other words, you will be enabled to lead a fulfilling life. Without your sleep, you will be miserable and make everyone who knows you miserable being around you. Without sleep you cannot share your best with those in your life stream, nor can you enjoy their company and your activities to the fullest.

With healthy sleep, you can accomplish whatever you want a lot faster, have a lot more fun doing it, and be a fun person to be with.

Remember my list of health problems, and the utter foggy misery I struggled with in just trying to get through the mundane tasks of my day? That is the hell to which you are bound if you don't fix your problem. Or worse; you could have a complete breakdown and get institutionalized. So the rewards easily outweigh any perceived sacrifice. Self-care is not a waste of time. In fact, it *saves* time. And money! No pills, doctors, operations, tests, confusion.

Also, this is not going to take forever. For some people with more minor sleeping problems, maybe a month or a few months. For people like me with severe insomnia, it is maybe a year or two. It took me about a year to be able to sleep a three to five hour stretch at a time. Another year or so to get to six or seven hours. This doesn't sound like much sleep, but you'll recall that I was sleeping sometimes as little as a few hours per week for four years. So three to five hours per night made me feel like a million bucks. I kid you not.

It is worth the time and the effort. *You* are worth it. It doesn't matter how you got here, to this low point. Let go of any guilt, shame, blame, and judgment about how you got here. If you waste brain cells obsessing about this, you are interfering with and actively preventing your healing. The only useful thing you can do now is move forward. How? Make the commitment to organize the rest of your life around trying to restore healthy sleep. That is your goal.

Do you want your life back? This single-minded focus is what it takes. Begin to simplify your life. When you have a medical crisis, that's what you have *to* do. Isn't it true that most of your circle is understanding and supportive when you're sick or injured and need a bit of space? They will respect your boundaries, so set them. They will respect your quiet resolve and your commitment to solving your own problems. They will admire you.

Put Yourself First by Simplifying Your Life

Take a look at your family life, your professional life, your social life and cut out the non-essentials. How can you simplify your personal and professional life?

- Reduce travel, long hours, and "wired" time.
- Cut out non-essential commitments. Don't spread yourself too thin. You can be an over-achiever again when your health problems are sorted out. Everyone will manage just fine without your giving 150%.
- Optimize your work time and tasks so that you can shorten your work day. Be a person who works smarter, not harder and longer.
- Don't be afraid to delegate and ask for help. Require more independence and self-reliance in children, and be willing to relinquish your control over every detail while you're under repair.
- Use commuting time and break time productively. Do some active meditations while driving, like sending kind thoughts to all the people that pass you and even to those who cut you off. This helps prevent road rage and keeps your mood light and bright. You can learn a language, listen to great tunes or audio-books, and interesting non-shock-jock news programs. Make it *you* time.
- Sneak in some extra exercise. If you can, get in some yoga or exercise during a break at work. A few minutes of stretching, a ten minute walk. If you work from home, give yourself permission to take short exercise breaks. The impact on your productivity and your back health is immediate.
- Commit to leaving your work at work, and not bringing it home with you. Turn off the phone and laptop if you can. Resist the temptation to check or answer your emails; they can wait.
- This goes for your head, too. Develop the discipline to be present in the moment and don't dwell on your work problems when

DR. FRANK R. SUTTON
216 1011 GLENMORE TR. SW
CALGARY AB
CANADA
T2V 4R6

TEL # 403 - 228 - 4211
FAX # 403 - 228 - 3362

Pureed

Chilled As

Hot & C

Pureed Carr

Pureed Wat

Puree

Break

you're not there. You can use a helpful mantra like "This is MY time. I focus it where I CHOOSE." You can say this to yourself when you find your thoughts straying back to work problems. As with any physical discipline, you have to practice doing this, and it gets easier with time and training.

- Set your boundaries gently and respectfully and stick to them. Others will follow your lead and do the same.

- Slow down a bit. Modern life has us in a constant rush. This approach to living makes us sick, mentally and physically, and there's no end to it unless you step back a bit. You don't need to move to a Tibetan monastery. Just take some reasonable measures. Remember to breathe deeply. Remember to be kind to strangers. Remember to talk less and listen more. As a contrast to my busier, manic days, I think of old Treebeard the Ent lumbering through Fanghorn Forest saying "Nothing is worth saying unless it takes a long time to say." (From The Lord of the Rings movie, The Two Towers.)

- Set limits about what happens at night, because you need peace and quiet. Don't sleep with your children. Don't sleep with your partner if he or she snores. Speak to everyone gently and respectfully about your needs and they will be grateful to help you.

- Cut out non-essential social activities and personal travel if it interferes with sleep training. Do the Australia trip next year. Postpone the Alaska cruise if you're worried about your roommate's snoring. Some house-moms I know are always exhausted from racing around from one social activity to the next. We have a habit of filling up our lives to the brim, thinking this will bring satisfaction and purpose. Don't worry about hurting your friends' feelings if you are less available; your circle of friends will appreciate your new goal, and respect your resolve. If they are true friends, they'll be waiting for you when you're done. Your kids will still thrive and get into good schools when they're older if you drive them around to fewer activities during the week..

- One of the most important ways to simplify your life is to pay no mind to the judgment and criticism of your family, colleagues, and doctors regarding your current medical crisis. Their opinion is none of your business. Why? For the simple fact that it takes valuable energy away from your new goal of restoring sleep health. You need to save every last bit of your strength for you, and not give it to strangers and people who can't help you and don't want to help you. Family can often be the biggest obstacle to major change and healing. Sometimes they prefer you to be suffering so they can manipulate you more easily. Often we listen to voices of authority, such as doctors, even when their advice counters our intuition. You need to tune out your family and the voices of authority that tell you sleeping pills can fix your insomnia, or you can't get your health back. There will always be people who like to criticize, and you don't have the bandwidth to handle it now. Time to close ranks to protect yourself. It's a life or death matter. Anyone who isn't helping doesn't have the right to have a voice in your process.

- Reduce your expectations of yourself. For busy working mothers, accept that your house will never look the way you want. You will never have enough time to do all the things you think you need to do. That is par for the course. It will change when your little ones are bigger. Anyone who criticizes you and your stained carpets can shove it. It's not your fault that they are ignorant enough to criticize you.

Simplifying your life doesn't mean you're underachieving or missing out on fun. Truly, as you reap the benefits of your authentic intention to restore healthy sleep, you will perceive these boundaries as luxurious self-pampering.

There is nothing on this planet that can keep me out of my bed when I decide I want to crawl in. If I want to do something extra special for myself, I don't buy a coffee or new shoes. I take a nap. If I'm not sleepy, but feel like a treat, I'll just lie down in a sunbeam and enjoy being horizontal, not worrying if I doze or not.

Before and After

Now. . . I usually fall asleep in less than thirty minutes and I stay asleep for at least four hours, usually about six hours.

Now. . . I usually have restful and deep sleep, even if it's not a lot.

Now. . . I don't jerk awake prematurely with a racing heart.

Now. . . I don't take any pills or medicines of any kind to assist with relaxation or sleep. No Tylenol PMs, valerian, melatonin, etc.

Now. . . I look forward to going to bed, instead of dreading it.

Now. . . I have normal, diverse dreams again, and I often remember them.

Now. . . I am able to fall asleep after being awakened by my children, even if it's more than a couple times per night.

Now, I enjoy life. I enjoy my work. I enjoy challenges and novelty and making plans. I'm able to have fun. I love being a mother. I can wash my hair and put on shoes. I can accept the challenges life hands me, and do my best to handle them with equanimity and creativity.

Summary

- Sleep deprivation is not a psychological problem that goes away by itself. You need to sort it out or it gets worse and you get really unhealthy in mind and body.
- Chronic sleep deprivation is a medical emergency. The health consequences of chronic sleep deprivation are diverse and severe.
- Take it seriously by making your sleep health a priority.
- Just like when you're sick, you need to simplify your life in order to restore good health.
- Sleep is powerful medicine. If you invest time in fixing yourself, you will experience great physical and psychological benefits. It is worth the time and effort.

2 YOU ALONE ARE RESPONSIBLE FOR FIXING YOURSELF

I know a few insomniacs who feel they can't go on any longer. I was one of them. Insomnia takes away your will to live. You'd rather die than spend another night sleepless, angry, and frustrated or another day dragging yourself through endless, exhausting tasks that no longer hold meaning or pleasure for you. You wake up not knowing how you are going to survive the day. You dread the nights because you fear not sleeping.

That's why sleep deprivation is such effective torture! It breaks your personality and your spirits very quickly.

When You Feel Bad, Your Body is Trying to Tell You Something!

Normal daily activities that most people take for granted are an unbearable burden for the insomniac. Let alone housework, a professional life or social activities. Every little thing feels so physically taxing. Getting dressed; getting undressed. Washing your face, scraping the snow off the car windshield.

I'd only bother changing my clothes when they stank of spit-up. Otherwise, same sweatpants and old T-shirt day and night. Covered the getup with a long coat if I was out in public.

23

You should have seen me trying to get a load of laundry up the stairs. You'd think I was running a marathon. I had to stop every couple stairs to rest my spinning head against the wall.

Why are simple, mundane activities so hard when you're not sleeping? The answer is very simple: when you feel this badly, your body is telling you something is very, very wrong. Think of it as powerful non-verbal communication. In this condition, you are so physically diminished that you can no longer sustain normal activity. Yet so many insomniacs persist in sticking to our aggressive schedules. We ignore the symptoms and fail to address the root problem.

Worse, often we interpret these remarkably clear signs of serious physical distress as some kind of psychological problem or weakness, some kind of character flaw:

"I'm not tough."
"I don't have what it takes."
" I'm lazy."
"There's something wrong with me, but if I ignore it, maybe it'll go away. "

None of this is true. You are not crazy. You are not lazy, or weak. And if you ignore your sleeping problems, they just get worse and you get sicker.

Nobody Can Understand Unless They've Experienced Insomnia or Sleeping Problems Personally

The thing is, unless you've experienced chronic sleep deprivation, you do not understand what this abyss is like. You are not able to have empathy and compassion for an insomniac. Hence many insomniacs don't have anyone to talk to, and if they do, they get blown off. You may find that those closest to you make you feel the worst.

During my most difficult months of sleeplessness, I rarely spoke of my despair and my darkest thoughts. I was too ashamed; I thought I was weak and selfish. My husband knew I wasn't sleeping at all, and he did lots of research for me on natural cures, but I didn't dare to speak to him of my cognitive and psychological disintegration. I was an angry, crabby cow. No one in my circle really knew why I was so difficult, but they sure were sick of it.

My other family members blew me off completely when I talked about being tired, let alone when I spoke of my deep depression. They couldn't stand my whining and complaining. They were busy with their own lives and wanted me to get over myself. There was no respect for my situation as a health crisis or emergency. They had absolutely no interest in helping me figure it out.

But even my long-suffering husband was unable to understand why I couldn't rationally problem-solve my sleeping issue. I sure could grumble, yell and cry, however. It was only after I was sleeping two or three hours a day that I had the mental capacity for rational thinking and problem solving. When sleeping just a few hours per week, I was not capable of such fundamental and normal activities like self-assessment, goal setting, action plans, execution of self-experiments, etc. I didn't know this either. I was living it, but I wasn't able to recognize just how cognitively impaired I had become.

If you are a long-term severe insomniac, your family's response to you may be similar. The lack of validation and understanding is crippling. Unfortunately, we often take their word for it, and instead of feeling sick, we feel crazy and stupid.

My family is made up of generally nice, decent, loving, helpful people. Perhaps this is what made their dismissal of my crisis so difficult for me. During one of my worst months, I had a lot of voiceovers to do, and no child care for my 2-year old and infant. They both slept poorly, so I just stayed up during the nights, nursing and pumping and consoling kids in between voiceovers, collapsing occasionally for a few moments on the sofa only to jerk awake with palpitations and sweats. I did this for weeks.

Occasionally my mom would come by during the day, and she'd drop hints about my seriously sub-standard housekeeping. "Your father doesn't like to visit because the mess stresses him out. You'll never get the damage deposit back the way you keep this house." When I tried to explain how I just couldn't handle it, she'd nod but keep the disgusted grimace plastered on.

My sister, who was my closest friend and confidante, dismissed me without a second thought, telling me repeatedly that every mother faced similar difficulties, that mine were no worse than anyone else's, that she hadn't had a good night's sleep either since having kids, and that I was simply lying about needing to work so much.

When I told them I wanted to kill myself and my children, my mom was embarrassed and promptly shushed me up. Her first words were, "Well, don't tell anyone!" My sister then suggested I take some

Omega-3 fish oil supplements.

Even now, it feels humiliating to admit just how messed up I was, and how little my family cared when I was in crisis. I am a driven, energetic person, and to have lost the will to live makes me feel like I've failed. In fact, I feel very vulnerable committing these words to paper for fear of being judged. For fear of being dismissed as a complete nutjob.

My family's inability to listen and understand made me feel really inadequate, like I was defective. I became even more self-critical, thinking I had made a major mistake by becoming a parent without having a stable income.

But mainly I was angry. Anger is an understatement, actually. I felt like a massive, rumbling volcano ready to blow out tons of poisonous gas and magma and engulf everything and everyone around me in the black haze of my rage. I was really stuck on the fact that my family refused to acknowledge the severity of my crisis. A lot of my thought and energy was poured into my rage.

In retrospect I see this was a complete waste of time and energy. Rage in this situation was not only ineffective, but counterproductive since it made me feel worse, and sleep even less. I shouldn't have given a damn about their opinion, because

1) It didn't help me sleep, and
2) It only slowed down my seeking help.

It took me a few more weeks to get post-partum support counseling. Another year before I gave up trying to control every moving part personally; I finally succumbed and put my kids in daycare.

Now, I'm glad we survived. I love life and more than anything I adore my amazing, beautiful children. I don't go five minutes without feeling a surge of gratitude. But I don't blame my family. I would never put the burden on them again of helping me sort out a big mess that I made. People can only see through the glasses they have. This is a limitation of human cognition. We are only able to perceive through the knowledge we've gleaned experientially. To expect anything different is a complete fantasy. If you expect otherwise you are expecting too much; you will end up disappointed and frustrated. Even though your family members love you, they cannot respect your medical emergency unless they have experienced it themselves.

Remind yourself not to take it personally. You cannot change human nature. It's a complete waste of time and energy that you need to conserve for yourself, to restore your healthy sleeping habits.

Doctors and Sleep Clinics Don't Help Much Either

Maybe you told your doctor you weren't sleeping well. He or she prescribed a sleeping aid and talked to you about lavender oil, no coffee after lunch, and no TV before bed. The pills don't help you sleep well, and they leave you groggy and thick during the day. But you're afraid to stop taking them in case you stop sleeping at all.

You go back a few months later and tell them how nervous and cranky you're getting, and that you're still not sleeping. Your dosage goes up and you get an anti-depressant prescription. Maybe a referral to a sleeping clinic.

You try out the clinic, full of high hopes. Finally, you think the experts are going to fix you. You like awake in a strange place, not sleeping. You get really stressed out from not sleeping and worrying about why. Then they put you on anti-anxiety meds to help manage the stress. After your two weeks, you go home, still not sleeping, now hooked on anti-anxiety medication.

Some sleep clinics are just drug trials for new sleeping pills, so maybe you've been a guinea pig without even knowing it. When you check out of a sleep clinic you often get more sleeping pills. I've known a few people who've attended sleep clinics (me included). We've all been frustrated by the lack of results. We all had drugs pushed on us, and no training in how to sleep.

Or maybe the only purpose of the sleep clinic was to diagnose sleep apnea. This refers to major pauses in breathing during sleep, and it is a very serious problem. You may have listened to your snoring father hold his breath for a long time in between big snores—this is an example of sleep apnea. It happens when the muscles around the airway relax during sleep, so then the airway collapses and blocks the intake of oxygen. Sleep apnea prevents you from going to deeper and REM sleep, because when oxygen levels in the blood drop, you come out of deep sleep to resume breathing. This can happen several times and hour, and you end up with little deep or "slow-wave sleep" and REM (dreaming) sleep. You might feel tired after getting many hours sleep but not know why. Most of the sleep clinics I've worked with can help diagnose this, but not provide the psychological training you need to teach yourself to sleep again if you don't have sleep apnea.

Now that you're back home, and even the professionals couldn't fix you, you're really worried. The clinic was the help of last resort. You waited for two years to get in there, or it cost you an arm and a leg at a private clinic. There's no other help out there. You're really stuck now. You're totally screwed, in fact. You can't take any more time off of work or away from your family. Now you're really anxious before going to bed, dreading the night, wondering if you will even fall asleep. Worrying about how you will make it through the next day if you don't get any rest. You take an extra sleeping pill, hoping it might help.

Thus traditional medical help can often be discouraging for the insomniac. When you're suffering from severe chronic insomnia you think you'll be stuck like that forever. It's unbearable.

No One Can Help You Except You

The truth of the matter is, no one can help you except you. Thirty years into the Age of Oprah Winfrey, this self-help mantra should ring familiar by now. You are responsible for solving this problem. You are the only one capable of solving this problem. You can't blame it on anyone else. The lack of validation from your family and the medical system makes you feel worse. You have to ignore them and stick to your guns.

I'm sure many post-traumatic stress disorder victims and prisoners-of-war who experience mental breakdowns find the same thing: those around them simply don't have the ability to comprehend what can happen to a brain, a personality, a spirit, when faced with the most extreme stresses people can endure.

In my diminished state I couldn't reason any of this out. I was only angry, angry, angry. Angry at myself for being a loser, and a failure, and one heck of a lousy mother. Angry at my family for not helping me in my hour of need, even though I'd have been there for them. Angry at the universe for doling me out such a crappy fate. I would obsess over it day and night.

What a ridiculous waste of my thoughts and my energy. Did it help me feel better? No, of course not.

But *why* not?

Well, when you're angry all the time, then every little thing makes you even more angry. My general agitation was increased tenfold. I'd lie awake at night seething with futile rage.

You may remember the Cherokee legend of the "Two Wolves";

this well-known story sums up the mind/body (emotions / hormones) connection in a most memorable way:

> An old grandfather, whose grandson came to him with anger at a schoolmate who had done him an injustice, said, 'Let me tell you a story. I too, at times, have felt a great hate for those that have taken so much, with no sorrow for what they do. But hate wears you down, and does not hurt your enemy. It is like taking poison and wishing your enemy would die. I have struggled with these feelings many times."
>
> He continued, 'It is as if there are two wolves inside me; one is good and does no harm. He lives in harmony with all around him and does not take offense when no offense was intended. He will only fight when it is right to do so, and in the right way. But the other wolf, ah! He is full of anger. The littlest thing will set him into a fit of temper. He fights everyone, all the time, for no reason. He cannot think because his anger and hate are so great. It is helpless anger, for his anger will change nothing. Sometimes it is hard to live with these two wolves inside me, for both of them try to dominate my spirit."
>
> The boy looked intently into his Grandfather's eyes and asked, 'Which one wins, Grandfather?" The Grandfather smiled and said, "The one I feed."

There are dozens of smart thinkers and writers who take up this topic using various spiritual and secular metaphors. Whether it's referred to as the law of cause and effect, the law of attraction, or "you are what you think", "you get what you give", etc, the meaning is the same: the more you dwell on thoughts that make you angry, the more angry you get.

I recommend that you read or listen to some of this material. I found it extremely helpful during my time of crisis. One of the earliest and most famous writers is Esther Hicks/Abraham, who wrote The Law of Attraction series. They have many straight-forward, quick and visual exercises you can jot down to help you let go of anger and blame. Most of the writers published by Hay House are superb, and one of them will fit your preferred perspective on this topic. Even better, there is a lot of listening material—either downloads of the radio shows from HayHouseRadio.com, or audio books. I listened to this kind of material all night long for years. More recently I started listening to classes by Jennifer Hadley; her work is very inspiring, and her voice and mannerisms are clear, pleasant, and easy to listen to (www.jenniferhadley.com).

Step #1: Stop Blaming Others

The first step in taking responsibility for your crisis and your healing is to stop blaming others. Don't waste any time and energy blaming your family or friends or job or doctor. Bemoaning that no one understands and wants to understand. Why nobody gives you a break. You may as well dump your life savings and two pints of blood in the toilet. Not only will you fail to get better, but waiting, expecting and blaming hampers your ability to solve your sleeping problem. You alone have the power and the ability to get your life back. You alone can help yourself. You are the only one who *can* help yourself.

How? You *simplify.*

Ask yourself: "Does blaming this person help me sleep? No. Does nursing my anger help me sleep?" No. So it's got to go. It's that simple.

If it seems more complex than this, it's because you don't want to make it simple. You don't want to let go of the anger. Remember my analogy about having a bad flu? There's nothing like vomit and diarrhea to clarify your next steps. You can't fight it; what for? You'll just make a big stinking mess everywhere and feel even worse. Instead, you go to bed with a bucket and you rest. You stay close to a toilet.

If you want your life back, you're going to have to practice making things simple. You need a very narrow focus. Like a computer, where all input and output is reduced to 1s and 0s.

"Does this help me sleep, yes or no?"

If yes, it stays. If no, out it goes. Bye-bye. Get rid of it. GROI.

I read somewhere that Madonna used to shout GROI when selecting what she liked from a photo shoot. GROI stands for **G**et **R**id **O**f **I**t.

GROI to blame. GROI to anger. You're in charge.

You must surrender that which does not help you sleep. Instead, you need to direct all your thoughts and energy to your single goal of restoring sleep health.

Even if you don't believe you can do it.

Even if you want someone else to help you because you you're afraid and you're tired and you're not used to doing hard things alone.

Even if you think you need someone else to help you because you don't have the mental and physical strength to do it alone, or you're just too busy to do it without help.

Even if you think other people should help you because they are related to you, or they love you, or you helped them when they needed help.

Even if you think someone else can help you because they are a medical professional.

Only you can restore your sleep health because you're the only one who lives in your body and knows what's going on. No one else has the knowledge required to make the adjustments it'll take to arrive at your personal solution. No one else is capable of making the personal investment required.

While I know lots of people with long term sleeping problems, I only know a handful of other people who have experienced severe chronic insomnia like I did. Some minds are already too broken by sleeplessness to pursue self-help. The road to healing may be longer and require medication / institutionalization if you have descended into a serious or psychotic depression. Institutions and medications don't treat the causes of insomnia, but they might prevent you from committing suicide.

If you can get stable enough on medication to start self-help, this is excellent. But then you need to wean yourself off drugs if appropriate. My experiences with friends, colleagues and family taking sleeping pills, anti-depressants, anti-anxiety medications, anti-psychotic medications and so on makes me think these don't help you solve your root problem. I'm not denying that some people really need medication to manage their conditions. However, there is a lot you can do to help yourself, also. For the most part, our own chemistry, which we adjust with food, thoughts, and exercise, is much more sophisticated, elegant and effective than anything we can get in a pill. Do what you can to help yourself and you will reduce your dependency on medication.

Some people are not self-confident enough by nature to trust that they alone are responsible for healing the body and mind. Most people have such little practice with mental discipline that they don't believe they accomplish this miracle. I felt this way, too. But anything is possible with focus and practice—with intention and appropriate action. Self-trust and self-confidence can also be developed this way.

Severe insomniacs will know that the line between sanity and insanity feels hazy and broad, and can be easily crossed. If you spend too much time "on the other side"—I used to call it the abyss, or the pit of despair—it will be that much harder to get healthy again. You need to start helping yourself before you get to this point.

And without a doubt, you will get to this point if you don't fix your insomnia. Remember, you are not crazy. You are sick, and you can heal yourself.

So, congratulations are in order if you have made it this far into this book. The ability to seek and commit to self-help is one sign of a healthy mind.

My Uncle's Story

When I finally discovered ways to treat myself, I decided it was important to share these ideas to help others in my situation, so they wouldn't have to do the research alone. I procrastinated for a while writing this book, being a busy working mom. But a recent family tragedy got me motivated to finally get this done. My uncle lost his wife (my aunt) to a difficult two-year battle with cancer. It was exhausting and terrifying; hope was constantly rolled out like a red carpet then pulled out from under their feet at the last minute. Unsuccessful surgeries, debilitating chemo, and a lot of pain and nausea. My aunt suffered long physical discomfort. Chronic pain and nausea are also very demoralizing. It was very hard for her family to watch her slip away so slowly and painfully.

During these two years my uncle experienced severe insomnia, sleeping only a couple hours every other night. He was institutionalized for a nervous breakdown within two weeks of her passing. We had no idea how to help him, because we couldn't make him sleep. We knew the problem was that he needed to sleep, then he'd be able to begin a period of healthy, "normal" grief. We thought psychiatric care would help him sleep. This was my family's first experience with mental health care. It is primitive. It is basically only pharmaceutical. He was prescribed anti-depressants, anti-psychotics and sleeping pills and received very little personal counseling. Yet during his three months in the hospital he continued to sleep terribly—just an hour or two every other night. His anxiety and paranoia grew. He was in a stupor all day trying to process the drugs which still couldn't help him sleep at night.

After three months he was released for the Christmas holiday, and was cut off cold-turkey from his anti-anxiety medication, to which he was now addicted. We didn't know anything about how the chemical cocktail of drugs worked; we could only see that they didn't seem to be working well. He committed suicide on his first night alone. He still wasn't sleeping at all.

Only later on did we find out that one can't quit anti-anxiety medications cold turkey; you need to wean yourself off in smaller and smaller doses. Often people are admitted to rehab centers for this purpose alone! We didn't know anything about the numerous pharmaceuticals administered, or how they worked. We didn't know these drugs had very bad side effects, such as rebound insomnia, paranoia, and withdrawal syndrome. Weren't the drugs supposed to help him, not make his insomnia and paranoia worse? We trusted the hospital to do the right thing.

We brought him to the hospital for help to get him sleeping again. They gave him a lot of pills that didn't help him sleep and that made his psychosis worse. The hospital staff were sorry that he was dead, but from their perspective there was no legal responsibility or negligence.

Of all his family members, I feel that I alone understood the agony of his years of sleeplessness. I did my best to talk to him and encourage him to put his rest first. With his wife of forty-five years wasting away right before his eyes, it was easier said than done. By this time, he'd already spent too much time in the insomnia abyss. At the time I was still barely sleeping at all and I had two children under age three to take care of, so my capacity for physical intervention was limited. We thought the hospital could sedate him for a couple days, and he would sleep and thus be rebooted. We didn't understand that's not how psychiatric care works. They haven't figured out how to help people with insomnia-induced breakdowns.

I learned during this time that once you have broken with reality, it's a long way back, and many people can't get back. The patients in the hospital were bleak caricatures of their former selves, wandering around in hospital gowns like broken prisoners from a 1950s film noir. There were a lot formerly successful, creative, driven, wealthy people in varying states of disintegration.

I learned it can happen to anyone, and how close I had come to that.

I was extremely discouraged by what I saw and heard in this hospital wing. I don't ever want to end up in such a place. I'll take a broken leg anytime over the nebulous, ambiguous terrain of a mental health problem.

You are helpless as you watch your loved one's personality disappear behind a heavy cloak of drugs. Mental health patients are often extremely unpleasant to work with, so you have to endure your loved one being treated with a cold lack of empathy and compassion by the staff. Frequently you can see how the staff despise their work, despise the patients, and despise family members also for challenging them to provide better care. You learn just how hard it is to get your groove back once your mind has been broken. You learn that anyone can become a crazy person under the right conditions, and it doesn't take very long, either.

That's why I stress the importance of dedicating your time and energy to restoring sleep health. You protect your house and your money and your car and your stuff by locking it up, right? You protect your body by wearing shoes and seatbelts and helmets and sunscreen. Sleep is how you retain and protect your sanity.

Once you're too far gone, all the king's horses and king's men can't put you back together again.

The Importance of Mental Self Care

The hopelessness and uselessness of psychiatric hospitalization in my uncle's case of insomnia-induced psychosis impressed upon me the importance of mental self-care. You don't need me to tell you that our society places a heavy emphasis on the physical. We are careful about what we eat. We read food labels and diet after Christmas to get back into our favorite jeans. We exercise to feel and look good. We wash our teeth and our skin and our sheets and clothes. We dye our hair when it's gray and get nipped and tucked and botox-ed to look young. We get a massage or visit a chiropractor or physiotherapist to fix a sore body. We go to the doctor for antibiotics if we have a bad ear infection.

Comparatively, we take much, much less care of our minds. We feel free to steep ourselves in anger, blame, worry, self-criticism and all sorts of self-destructive thoughts. We are rigorous in keeping our bodies fed with food, physically exercised with all sorts of practices, cleaned with showers, soaps, deodorants and perfumes, but we take almost no care to nourish and clean our minds and spirits. Once you have developed a practice that helps you take care of your mind and spirit, you will realize just how crazy it is to expect your mind to function well without any maintenance and care.

Our relentless mind chatter and chronic criticism of ourselves and others can be self-destructive on many levels, but the only aspect that concerns me here is that it doesn't let you sleep.

If something doesn't let you sleep, it is destructive and it has to go. GROI. Get rid of it!

How many people do you know that incorporate daily mental self-care into their routine? Not a single person in my circle does, and I travel with a lot of new-age hipsters. They smoke weed, have coffee breaks, complain to friends, take vacations in Mexico. Not even everyone in my spiritual group meditates regularly or even frequently. It is really hard to turn down the volume of our noisy, critical, judgmental minds. From my experience with the few severe insomniacs in my acquaintance, and with those I know who have sleeping problems, not a single one has a practice of mental self-care. I didn't either.

Why is it so unnatural for us to take care of our minds? The thing is, it's not like it takes much time. It's about attitude, not effort. So what's the hold up?

Many of us come from cultures and religions which lead us to believe that unless we're tormented by guilt or pelted by constant criticism, we run the risk of underachieving. Only by focusing on our failure do we get ahead.

In my Italian village, if you ask people how they are, no one dares admit they are doing 'ok'. Any expression of contentment and gratitude is tantamount to hubris and, like a lighting rod, is likely to attract a strike from angry gods above.

For men, the practice of mental self-care is that much more difficult. Younger men may be more familiar and comfortable with the discourse of mental self-care, but for many older men, it's a foreign language. If you talk about this concept with, for example, my father, who is an old-fashioned Italian immigrant in his early 60s, he'll have no idea what nonsense you are on about. Even my husband, who's a real tough-guy from Russia in his early 40s, can't relate to this discourse. My uncle was the same way. If you stop mind-churning, or even if you talk to your friends about your problems, you are just too soft and you don't have enough to do. My dad's idea of mental self-care is a hard day's work followed by a warm meal at the table, quiet kids and grandchildren, the six-o'clock news and a nap in his favorite chair. Nothing wrong with this; in fact, this is a great way for men to regenerate testosterone. But when you're not sleeping well, more is required.

The anthropology of this issue is more complex than I will delve into here, but suffice it to say that we have a lot of built-in resistance to the practice of mental self-care. Plus, even here in the "first world" we are only about two generations removed from subsistence living. As recently as the Great Depression most people struggled to eke out the basics of human survival—food, shelter, warmth. So we don't have much practice, either, at taking care of our minds. We've been too preoccupied with not starving or freezing. In my family, it's just one generation ago: my parents, and my uncle, grew up in a decimated post-WWII southern Italy. They endured severe poverty and hunger in the 1950s, and eventually they immigrated to Canada as teenagers in the late 1960s.

What do I mean by mental self care? What should you be doing if you want to sleep better? I did mention meditation earlier, which is very helpful and I highly recommend it. I'll talk about it a bit more later on. But mental self-care for insomniacs is a lot more than this. I wasn't able to meditate when I wasn't sleeping much; I simply didn't have the ability to focus. You have to start somewhere easier.

Step #2: Let Go of Toxic Thoughts

I believe there are two key steps, your cornerstones for repairing your mind. Step one is accountability: accept that you alone are responsible for helping yourself, and that it's ok that no one can help you as much as *you* can help you. Stop and pat yourself on the back, darling, because that is a huge accomplishment. Now you're ready for step two.

Step two is letting go of toxic thoughts. Toxic thoughts are things that make you feel fear, worry, shame, blame, guilt, rage, anger, resentment, regret, and more. Letting go of toxic thoughts is absolutely fundamental for the insomniac.

I call the thoughts "toxic" not because they are "negative," or because they attract bad stuff into your life, or make you feel worse, or because you are what you think, etc. All this is true of course, but for the purposes of this book I pronounce them toxic merely because they keep you awake:

The more you think about stuff that makes you angry, resentful, guilt-ridden, ashamed, worried, fearful, frustrated etc., the less likely you are to sleep.

You can take lots of sleeping pills, stop coffee, spend suitcases of money on a sleep clinic and psychologists and therapy, and spritz lavender on your pillow for the rest of your life but if you're stewing in the middle of the night over your issues you will not be able to restore healthy sleep. No way. Especially if you're a woman because we really enjoy stewing in our emotions.

It is ironic that the best solutions for health problems are often free, for most people. But they are not easy, until you are willing:

Want to lose weight? Eat less.

Sore back? Stretch more. Work less. Change your mattress or chair.

Feel sad? Count your blessings and take time to do stuff that you like.

Our lack of willingness has manifested as the multi-billion dollar health and pharmaceutical industries. So not only is your intention worth billions of dollars but it is extremely powerful: once you direct your intention to fixing your problems instead of complaining about your misery, you can take off like a rocket.

Letting go of your toxic thoughts is not easy, until you are willing. When you become willing, then it becomes easy. So, how do you develop the *willingness* to let go?

You have to want to sleep more than you want to hold your grudge. You can become willing, with practice.

Some people just refuse to do it. Thus they choose self-destruction over healing. But you can become willing, with practice.

People carry a lot of baggage. Often we were born right into a big pile of it. Releasing anger and blame and regret and resentment and guilt and shame and worry and fear and rage and so on takes constant attention until you build up the discipline of not thinking those thoughts. In fact, you have much more time when you let these thoughts go. These toxic thoughts take up a lot of bandwidth in our brains, much more than we realize. When they're gone you have all that extra bandwidth available for yourself and your healing.

Mental Discipline Takes Training

Letting go of your toxic emotions at night, when you should be sleeping, is a mental discipline. Whether physical or mental, a discipline requires exercise. You have got to practice. Let's say you dislike physical activity, but your doctor told you to exercise. You don't want to spend the money on a gym membership. So you start out with a slow walk. It's nice out, and you enjoy the down time. Months pass and you're walking faster. Soon you're looking forward to your daily walk because it's fun to see who's out and you enjoy the sunset. One day you break into a jog for ten seconds. It felt great to move so fast, but it was a bit jostling and tiring. You walk a bit more and then you try it again. This time it's easier.

You're so excited that you go again in a couple days, and this time you're able to run for a bit longer. You feel a huge surge of pride in your accomplishment. You feel inspired. You are happy. That happiness fuels your efforts next time you go. Soon you're enjoying it just for the physical rush it gives.

Mental disciplines work just like this. At first it's not exciting or easy, but your investment and enjoyment grows because it feels good and you feel better.

When I was a teenager, my mom always had Oprah or Dr. Phil on while we were preparing supper, and I remember Dr. Phil lecturing to squabbling married couples—"Do you want to be RIGHT or do you want to be HAPPY?"

You have to choose.

Unfortunately, I think most people want to be right AND happy.

We think we need to be right to be happy. We are often not willing to compromise. We're often not able to identify how to compromise.

For the insomniac, the questions relate to your medical emergency, which simplifies your life and lays forth the choices involved in compromising:

Do you want to be healthy?

Do you want to be sane?

Do you want to be alive in five years? Or would you rather noodle your resentments and regrets at night instead of sleeping?

It comes down to that binary choice. If you choose to nourish your anger and blame, then you do not heal your mind very quickly. In fact, you might lose your mind. Certainly, you will not restore healthy sleep anytime soon.

You choose: you are the boss.

Feed Your Mind Well So You Can Learn to Sleep Again

Maybe you are so miserable and exhausted right now that you don't care if you're alive in five years. I get it. I spent *years* feeling too tired to live another day. Maybe it doesn't feel like you are in charge. Maybe you feel like the victim of so many unkind, ungrateful people. Please keep reading and try anyway, because three years ago I was you. All I needed was some sleep, and so do you. We think in this fatalistic, paranoid way because we can't sleep. This is your misperception of reality, which gets corrected when you're sleeping.

If your stomach is really sore, do you eat steak and kidney pie slathered in gravy and melted cheese? Nope. In fact, you might not eat at all until you feel better. You might just drink fluids or juice. Or eat foods that are light and easy to digest. The same principle applies to your mind: when you are in the insomnia abyss, don't load yourself up at night with thoughts that make you angry and fearful. Instead, you must practice "feeding" your mind the light thoughts that are easy to digest!

This doesn't mean you're sticking your head in the sand or the clouds. You'll have plenty of opportunity to direct useful thought and action to solving your problems. Just not when you're supposed to be asleep! With good sleep, your ability and efforts will have that much more potency. Without rest, it takes longer and it's harder.

But how can I stop worrying?

But do you realize how badly he hurt me?

Everyone is laughing at me. How can I hold my head up?

My life is ruined.

This job just takes such a toll on me; I can't relax.

I will never recover from this.

Easy for you to talk. You're not about to lose your home.
Your wife is not dying.
Your son wasn't arrested.
You weren't raped.
You're not being bullied.

I hear lots of "buts". Yeah. Welcome to being human. Birthing, relating, surviving, aging, suffering, dying: none of this is easy and problem free, for anyone. We make it a lot harder and less fun by noodling over it at night instead of sleeping.

Being human leaves muddy residue. It's up to you to wash it off, every day. Several times a day if necessary. If you want to teach yourself to sleep again, this is what it takes.

For me, the middle of the night used to be such an awful time of blackness and despair. I just couldn't get free of my head. I felt like there was a sledgehammer in there pounding my brain into pemmican. Usually about 4am, an abyss of panic and fear would open up. Issues I could weather during the day became completely insurmountable. I just ached to die, to disappear. You hear that you shouldn't stay in bed once you can't sleep; you should get up and move around a bit, read on the sofa. I was afraid to get up, because if I moved I was afraid that I'd kill myself. I spent about three years like this, afraid to move at night in case I killed myself.

Yet even in those darkest moments, I made the choice for healing because I chose not to move. There was some seed of hope left, and thus I chose not to move. If I had access to the information I share with you now, I could have taken the high-speed gondola out of the abyss instead of crawling out on all fours blindfolded and mewling. So keep reading!

The bottom line is, you must choose. Do you want to heal yourself or not? You cannot teach yourself to sleep again if you don't make an effort to surrender resentment, regret, worry, fear, blame, anger, rage, shame, guilt, and all those toxic emotions. You have to choose. Remember, your intention is very powerful--it's even worth billions of dollars!

Your intention is the most powerful thing you have!!

Why do you need to let go of toxic thoughts?

Because they keep you up at night more than anything. They make body chemistry that keeps you awake. To help your body sleep, you have to control your thoughts. And you are the only one who can control your mind. Nobody can help you do this.

You alone rule your mind. You alone must rule it.[2]

Some things you don't have control over: the actions of others, in public or at work, or even in your home. But your mind—this is the one thing you have absolute mastery over, because nobody else is in there.

When you find your mind straying to toxic thoughts at night, use a safe word or phrase. I used to say, "banish it." I've heard other words used, like delete, cancel, get rid of it, begone, junk, flush, bye-bye.

Even if you're already ten minutes into the fantasy monologue where you're letting the mean co-worker or your passive-aggressive mother-in-law have it. Just stop wherever you're at, and banish the thought.

I used to say to the toxic thought: "You are banished, now and for all time."

I've got a couple visualizations that were very helpful for me. If you are a visual person, you will resonate with this way of doing things. I used to close my eyes and see a computer desktop, with folders I could sort as neatly as I liked. I enjoyed "tidying" my mind, because, running a business from home with two busy toddlers underfoot, often my house and my work were in total disarray and chaos. This activity helped alleviate anxiety about those messes. Each time the toxic thought arose, I'd banish it and see myself dragging it into the computer recycle bin. Then I'd empty the bin and permanently delete the thought.

Of course my mind circled back to it three seconds later and I'd do the same thing again and again and again. Then I'd get sick and bored and frustrated of that and try something else. I visualize a nasty, stinking, hot, cockroach-infested dumpster. I'd dump my thought into this epitome of grossness. I'd indulge myself in recoiling at the repulsive filth of the dumpster and ask myself, "Do I really want to put that maggoty, festering sludge back in my head? Come on, don't do it. Yuck." Sometimes this made me giggle, and take myself less seriously. Humor is a great way to change your mental channel, as we will discuss in a subsequent chapter of this book.

So I'd do this, dozens of times an hour, and hour after hour. Banish thoughts, over and over. Sometimes I'd doze, wake up

---

[2] A Course in Miracles, Lesson 236. Published by the Foundation for Inner Peace.

enraged, banish the thoughts, lie awake. Read a bit. Deal with the kids. Repeat. Lie awake. Trash the thoughts. Repeat. Repeat. Repeat. Repeat.

Sometimes I'd get really impatient and frustrated having to do it so many times. Why wasn't I developing the automatic ability to filter my thoughts? Why was I holding this resentment so tightly? What did I value so much about my toxic thoughts that they were more important than my sleep? What was wrong with me that I couldn't let go?

So then I'd visualize myself connected to two giant pipes, about eight inches wide each. One was sucking the black poison out of my brain. It writhed and twisted like a massive anaconda as it sucked my unforgiving, mean, hateful thoughts out and out, It took my mean, paranoid, angry thoughts back to the void where such useless crap belonged. The other pipe delivered blue-white light to my mind at the same time. I'd visualize it comfortably searing through the wasteland of my brain, cleaning and tightening my wiring, and restoring me back to the innocent, enthusiastic person I once was, crystallizing me into a shiny diamond.

This might all sound too mystical, but this last visualization was extremely helpful for me. Just a minute of this visualization took the edge off a migraine like nobody's business.

They say it takes seventeen days to make a habit, and about six weeks for children. So practice! What have you got to lose? It's free. No bad side-effects. And the results are immediate.

I also have positive affirmations taped to places that I frequent the most. Car dashboard, kitchen window above the sink where I wash dishes, piano, computer, bathroom mirror. Desk, work notebook. I often would write on my arm with a fat black sharpie so I couldn't miss it:

I let go of this thought because it no longer serves me. I alone rule my mind.

So What Do I Think About, Then?

You may have spent so long nursing your resentments and guilt and worry that when you shut them off, you can't find anything to think about. Anger, rage, shame, guilt, blame, worry, and fear take up way too much of our mind-chatter. For me, 100% of my mind-chatter was hijacked by anger, regret and worry. Once I tried to banish them, then what? The hole they left was massive. I felt lost without my anger. It was so much easier to dwell on anger than to do something constructive. I had energy when I was angry. It was the only time I could do anything quickly.

Also, I felt I wasn't being honest and realistic if I wasn't cataloguing my gripes. Reliving my anger and obsessing over my problems was how I proved I wasn't in denial. I felt that in order to be truthful, I needed to review and relive these dramas incessantly. Responding to anger brought me a sense of urgency and purpose; it gave me drive and passion.

We enjoy drama. We get used to it. We get off on it. That's why it takes so long to let go of our toxic thoughts. They bring a lot of meaning to our lives. That's was my experience, and that's why I was so slow to develop the ability to filter my negative thoughts out automatically. My intention wasn't lined up 100%. I still valued my toxic thoughts enormously because they gave me energy and purpose. This was why I had to self-correct a hundred plus times an hour.

So what do you do in the middle of the night if you're not supposed to think angry thoughts? What can you put in that big mad hole? Thinking about *nothing* is just too hard for the insomniac; you don't have the ability to concentrate anymore and hence it is nearly impossible to empty your mind.

Sometimes my kids ask me if there really is magic. I usually say, "yeah, just not like on TV." But that's actually not true. We earthlings have an incredible alchemical agent available to everyone, all the time, and for free. It's called gratitude.

There's a reason your grandmother told you to count your blessings. Gratitude is the most remarkable medicine we have in our thought system. There's a chemical reason why you feel so good when you count your blessings: it's how you push your brain's happy button. I'll explain exactly how this works in chapter four. Instead of cataloguing your gripes in the middle of the night when you should be sleeping, start making lists of what you are grateful for.

You can transform this:

"I'm so tired and I've got to do all that cleaning or it will never get done and there is nobody to help me and everyone just keeps making more of a mess that they expect me to clean up and how am I going to make money when I'm so tired and everything is so expensive?"

Into this:

> "I'm grateful that who I truly am isn't measured by how many dirty dishes I have and how sticky my floor is. I am grateful that I am much, much more than this. I'm grateful that I can choose when to clean it. I'm grateful that I feel great when my kitchen is clean. I'm going to take a few moments to appreciate my work when I'm done cleaning. I'm grateful for the food I have prepared in and on the dishes, food that nourishes my family and I. I'm grateful for my abundance—for this home that keeps my family and I warm and safe. For the food we share together. I'm grateful that I have dishes and utensils for preparing food. I'm grateful for what I have. I'm grateful for my family and for having made a home where my children feel comfortable and safe to explore and try new things. I'm grateful for the opportunity to care for my family. I'm grateful for the uniqueness brought to the mix by each of us. I'm grateful that we're different and quirky. I'm grateful that we've come together this lifetime to learn and live and love together. I'm grateful for this time awake to express my gratitude about my family and my abundance. I'm grateful for this mattress which feels pretty good. I'm grateful for these blankets which are really soft. I'm grateful for the clean air that I'm breathing now. I'm grateful for the quiet and stillness of the night."

You see how quickly gratitude magnifies and multiplies? It's like Rumplestilskin, spinning gold out of straw. Instead of resenting your dirty house and endless chores, and fuming at your spouse for being so unhelpful, focus on how wonderful it is to have a house, dishes, enough food to eat, and children and a partner who are strong, healthy and playful enough to make a mess in it. You can do this to any situation.

Gratitude can quickly encompass any complaint and totally flip the table on foul night-time thinking. In our forward-thinking, future-focused world, we feel that if we stop to appreciate the present, we're not making progress toward our future goals. As a species we've built up the habit of complaining instead of counting our blessings. The middle of the night is when your darkest thoughts creep out from under the bed and stare you down. Gratitude is the way to prevent them from becoming permanent squatters in your head. Gratitude fills the night-time emptiness and replaces worry, despair and anger. If you want to teach your mind to sleep again, this is the way.

We've got a long history of remarkable teachers who felt the same way. Jesus. Buddha. Gandhi. Martin Luther King. Mother Teresa. Thich Nhat Hanh. All of these teachers faced great physical hardship, and they still believed and practiced it.

On the very day I that started practicing gratitude in the middle of the night, I was able to fall back asleep after about 30 minutes of heart-pounding. Within a couple weeks I became able to sleep two or three hours in a row. Before this time, I had begged and begged the universe for some release from the strain of being inside my brain. I had been listening to helpful meditations for years, but sometimes they got on my nerves and I'd tune them out. Especially if I was mad about not sleeping. Gratitude was exactly what I had been looking for. It was the instant antidote to frustration. For me, this was nothing short of a miracle. Usually if my heart-pounding started, there was no more sleep for me at all, even if it was as early as midnight. Once gratitude stopped my heart from racing, I was able to listen to the meditation material and find benefit from it.

Why was this a miracle?

Because just a little more sleep changes a lot. It means everything.

When I started sleeping two or three hours in a row per day, there was an incredible and instantaneous improvement in every bodily function, physically and psychologically.

- No suicidal and homicidal thoughts and urges. The worst of post-partum depression was instantly evaporated, without pills, therapy, anything. Just a wee little bit of sleep, two to three hours in a row per night.
- Fewer headaches, with diminished severity. I used to have crippling migraines for days at a time. No night-time headaches.
- More steady hands; no more vertigo and no more nausea.
- Resting heart rate quite a bit lower. Fewer instances of racing heart during the day and night.
- No confusion regarding visual and aural inputs; it was a lot easier to drive without nervousness.
- Decreased sensitivity to light, sounds and smells.

45

- Enormous decrease in daytime rage and anger. I was much less crabby!
- Restored ability to handle routine tasks without physical fatigue and emotional exhaustion.
- Increased patience and problem-solving ability when handling challenges.
- Increased experience of pleasure in life.

So what was I grateful for? As a mother of young children, what I'd do is think about how much I loved my children. I'd visualize their beautiful soft faces lively with play or quiet in repose, breathing slowly and peacefully in slumber. Instead of cataloguing my woes, I'd focus on their cuteness in minute detail, taking my time, because I had all night to do it. I had accepted that I was likely to be awake all night, and might as well enjoy this moment. I'd see their hair and little kid-noses; their squishy legs and bums and fine skin; I'd imagine them hugging me or kissing me, and revel in the bliss of their soft touch.

That doesn't mean they didn't drive me bonkers half the time. My kids are busy daredevils. I had to childproof everything under six feet in my house and keep all the chairs locked in bedrooms because the boys climbed everywhere. There were plenty of phones and jewelry and remote controls and cutlery down the toilet. Hand cream and soap sprayed all over the walls and floor, all the time. Markers and crayons and food coloring in the carpet and all over the walls and mirrors and windows. Endless whining and tantrums. Zero time for myself. No sense that anyone appreciated any of my hard work. Some days I spent hours changing diapers and washing poop out of clothes. In the wintertime my hands were so raw and chafed I couldn't get the poop out of the cracks in my fingertips without a toothpick. I don't think I had the toilet or tub to myself for about three years straight.

But during the night I chose to focus on only the good stuff and I banished the rest. The more you do it the easier it gets. Not only with my children, but with the other issues that bothered me. I chose to appreciate how nice it was that I could give my mom some mending and she'd do such a terrific job. Or that my sister threw great dinner parties, and my dad bought only the best meat for our weekly Sunday barbeque. Or that my job gave me the independence to care for my children myself, and work from home.

Why does thinking grateful thoughts get easier with practice? A very well known Buddhist monk, Thich Nhat Hanh, sums it up in a gardening analogy. He says we need seeds that are beautiful, healthy and strong enough to help us during difficult moments:

> Consciousness exists on two levels: as seeds and as manifestations of these seeds. Suppose we have a seed of anger in us. When conditions are favorable, that seed may manifest as a zone of energy called anger. It is burning and makes us suffer a lot.... Every time a seed has an occasion to manifest itself, it produces new seeds of the same kind. If we are angry for five minutes, new seeds of anger are produced and deposited in the soil of our unconscious mind during those five minutes. That is why we have to be careful in selecting the kind of life we lead and the emotions we express....Every time we practice mindful living, we plant healthy seeds and strengthen the healthy seeds in us....If we plant wholesome, healing, refreshing seeds, they will take care of the negative seeds, even without our asking them. To succeed, we need to cultivate a good reserve of refreshing seeds.[3]

It's the practice, the *habit* of nourishing the seeds that makes the difference. The practice is the water, the sunlight and the dirt that enables the seeds to grow. If you have a habit of complaining and cataloguing resentments, then these are your seeds, and they grow into thorny weeds that give you no relief. If you plant seeds of gratitude, your yield is much more useful. Chemically, this is because gratitude releases, and also helps you make, your happy hormones and neurotransmitters (the latter are chemicals you make, that work inside your brain). Without these happy chemicals, you feel terrible. With these happy chemicals, you can manage the ups and downs of life with strength of purpose and patience.

Some soldiers with sleeping problems that I've spoken with made their strongest bonds with their comrades during deployments. My husband was a soldier in the Russian army and special forces, and for him also, the most powerful relationships of his life were forged during these years. The bonds with his comrades are much stronger than his bond with me or even our children. So if you are a soldier, you can visualize your best buddies; catalog their quirks and

---

[3] Thich Nhat Hanh, <u>Peace is Every Step</u> (Bantam Books, 1991), 73-77.

vulnerabilities and innocence and soft spots. Men release their happy hormone, testosterone, when they feel good about their accomplishments, so take some time to catalog what you are proud of, and what you enjoy about your work, or about your efforts.

As soon as I found myself dwelling in anger on my husband for not wanting to help with the kids, I banished these thoughts to my stinky dumpster and would focus instead on what he did bring to our household:

> I am grateful to my husband for the help he does provide. Scraping the windshields. Shoveling the snow. Fixing the toilet. These little things are hard for me and save me a lot of time and hassle.

In any situation that is bothering you, pick out what is working well, and put your energy there. Here are just a few examples:

- I am grateful that my boss makes herself available to listen to me.
- I am grateful that my wife takes pride in the cleanliness of our home.
- I am grateful that my daughter has a bright and bubbly personality and likes to talk to people.
- I am grateful my son is independent and healthy and curious about the world.
- I am grateful that I can help people everyday at my job.
- I am grateful my parents were healthy and strong for so long.
- I am grateful to have a lot of time alone to focus on my health, and to do things that I like.
- I am grateful to have people around me all the time because I don't like being alone.
- I am grateful that I have a house to live in that is already paid for.

I heard a story recently about a mother from South Sudan. Fleeing the civil war, she and her five children walked without food or water to a refugee camp in Kenya. The journey was thirty days. Single mothers and their families were frequently victims of sadistic violence by highwaymen and soldiers. Some of her children were so near death that at some point the mother was forced to abandon them on the road, so she could carry her stronger children to the camp. After the long walk, she arrived at the camp only to find that women and children remained terribly vulnerable to rape, murder, kidnapping and theft, and couldn't muscle their way to any food or water.

This is a person with problems.

I am so haunted by this story that whenever I find myself lapsing into self pity, it comes to mind. Any problem I have could never come close to this. Contemplate the suffering of this woman, and then dare to tell yourself that you can't find ten thousand things to be grateful for. I've heard it said that if you can be grateful for seven things each day, you can stave off depression. That's another example of how much thought and energy we invest in noodling over problems. We practice comparatively little investment in being grateful for what is working out well.

If you think you can't find anything to be grateful for, there's a reason: you are really out of practice. You've probably practiced very hard at complaining and cataloguing your woes, though. I sure did. Science tells us that our emotions work to rewire our brain: when we are chronically angry, this is how we stimulate ourselves, and we require ever more anger to feel the same stimulation. Think of the rush you get when you are filled with righteous anger. It feels good to have such a jolt of passion about something, doesn't it? It's clear and strong:

- That jerk just cut me off. What a stupid prick. What makes him think he's better than me, because he drives a big truck and my car is crappy, old and slow?
- She has no idea how much she hurts me, and how much I do for her anyway.
- My children are so ungrateful. I have given them everything and they don't give a damn. They still treat me with such disrespect.
- That hospital killed my uncle. I won't rest until those doctors lose their licenses.
- Who are the rapists and bullies that drove this teenage girl to suicide? They should be humiliated publicly if the police won't put them in jail.

If the only time you feel clear and strong is when you're in the throes of a righteous anger and blame, then you are addicted to your own drama. Think about how much of your thoughts are dedicated to anger, fear, shame, blame, regret, rage, guilt and more. For me, during my time in the insomnia abyss, it was 100%. This is a sign that I was seriously out of practice counting my blessings, and chemically addicted to my ideas of suffering. This is certainly not healthy, but in our society, it is perfectly normal. Unfortunately, this means you will keep making drama so you can get the jolt or rush.

For this reason, it is important to cultivate the practice of gratitude. You will literally change your brain chemistry, and I talk more about this in the fourth chapter of this book. If you are really depressed and honestly can't think of anything to be grateful for, you are not alone. Begin by contemplating the constants in life, the aspects of our existence that are not riddled with doubt. This is a technique recommended by famous Buddhist teachers. Thich Nhat Hanh might call it cultivating seeds of wisdom, and Venerable Dwani Ywahoo might call it energizing the ideal:

- The sun rises, and sets.
- The tides go in and out.
- The seasons come and go and come again.
- The rain is followed by sun.
- My heart beats.
- My breath goes in, and out.
- The planets orbit around the sun. Our solar system orbits around the galaxy's center. Our galaxy orbits around something else, something even more massive.
- There are more stars in the heavens than grains of sand on earth.

From there, start with the small things in your life that you are grateful for, like your senses and your breath. Be grateful that you can see, hear, smell, taste and/or feel, and think of something you like to look at, or smell, etc. A fragrant flower is something that reaches many of our senses. It is beautiful, extremely intricate in design and engineering. The smell is glorious, more wonderful and enchanting than any perfume made by people. The texture of the petals is soft and exquisite. Feel the petals between your fingertips; allow the heavenly fragrance to glide up your nostrils, and marvel at its magnificent design.

Chronic pain that keeps you awake is very difficult. It is hard to focus away from pain, and every time you move, you wake yourself up. It is exhausting to be in chronic pain. It is also demoralizing. When you're in chronic pain, it's more important than ever to focus on what you are grateful for. Catalog the parts of your body that are working well. Your heart is pumping strongly. Your feet and toes that let you walk. Your hands that allow you to eat and handle things, touch and feel and know so much of the world. Make a list during the daytime so that you can read it to yourself at night. Get someone to help you, if you can't think of anything to write down. You can ask to know the life lesson from your pain, and ask for the grace and patience to navigate your condition more easily.

When you're awake in the middle of the night, you need something to think about instead of your problems, and if you connect to something larger outside yourself, or smaller than yourself, it is easier to navigate out of our natural yet often purposeless and harmful narcissism. While it might seem silly or a waste of time to think about galaxies or petunias, you need to think about something other than your problems at night so you stop making the stress hormones that keep you awake and make you sick. You can try pills that don't work and shorten your life span, you can scream at your family and stew in your suffering, or you can think about things and people that activate your own natural sleeping and healing chemicals. You get to choose. You are the boss. You are the only one who can make it happen. Like with any exercise or skill, when you practice your willingness and ability grow.

Even though I'm sleeping well now, if I happen to wake up in the middle of the night, I will still tally things I am grateful for until I fall back asleep. The first few lines go like this:

- I am grateful for gratitude.
- I am grateful I know it works.
- I am grateful to be here.
- I am grateful gratitude brought me here.
- I am grateful the air is clear and clean.
- I am grateful I can breathe easily.
- I am grateful it is quiet and still.
- I am grateful the sun will be up in a few hours.
- I am grateful the moon is overhead now, and the stars.

If there is something that's bothering me, I will identify how I can be grateful for it also:

51

- I am grateful for having gotten stuck in the snow and caused a traffic jam. I'm grateful it helped me realize I'm not patient enough with myself, I worry too much about what others think, and I need to take better care of my tires in the winter. I'm grateful for this reminder, and that nothing more serious happened.
- I am grateful that I'm sensitive because otherwise I may not have learned all these important life lessons in self-reliance.
- I am grateful that woman yelled at me in the grocery store because I had a chance to keep calm and collected when it mattered.
- I'm grateful that woman yelled at me in the grocery store because it helped me see I'm not as calm and collected as I'd like to be when it really matters. I'm grateful for this knowledge and will try harder next time to walk my talk.
- I'm grateful I made this mistake, because that's what it took for me to learn what I really wanted.
- I don't understand right now why she isn't returning my calls / why I got sick / why they don't want to spend time with me, but I am grateful there are lessons in all my experiences and I am grateful that I will at some point soon have clarity as to why this is happening.
- I'm grateful that my work environment is so energetic and busy. I'm grateful for what I'm able to contribute, and I'm grateful for the contributions of others also. I'm grateful for the ability to step back when I need to and not engage with others' busy-ness.

The active practice of gratitude is the key item in mental self-care. For every worry and problem, flip it on its head to discover the blessing and put your energy into gratitude. If you're not used to meditating, you'll find that this is a lot easier. It's a lot more effective and powerful than pills. It was my first lifeline out of the abyss of insomnia. It is a tool I still use daily and will use for the rest of my life.

And now, my young jedi, you are ready. You have accepted that you alone are responsible for sorting out your sleep health. The most important part of this responsibility means releasing those thoughts that keep you awake at night, and filling that space with gratitude instead.

This is utterly transformative and powerful because it means the difference between *no sleep* and *some sleep*. You are now more than ready to begin your journey to sleep health.

SUMMARY

- When you feel bad, this is your body's way of telling you something is wrong. Don't ignore it and keep clinging to the status quo.
- Unless your doctors, family, friends and colleagues have experienced sleep deprivation / insomnia, they cannot understand how bad you feel. This can be very discouraging and slow down your healing.
- Don't be ashamed. You are not defective. You are not crazy. You are sleep-deprived and it's a real, physical problem.
- Only you can help yourself. You have to cowboy up and own this problem. There is no alternative.
- Sleep equals sanity. Chronic sleep deprivation can create psychological problems that are hard to fix. You have to help yourself before it is too late.
- Just a little extra sleep goes a long way to making you feel better.
- Mental self-care is not natural for people, but is very important to restoring sleep health. The payback is enormous; it is easily worth the effort.
- Banish blame, anger and resentment and other toxic thoughts in the night because they make it harder to sleep.
- Instead, count your blessings because this helps you make your body's natural happy chemicals for sleeping, healing and stress-relief, and these are more powerful than pills.
- Banish / Gratitude gets easier with practice, but the benefit to your sleep manifests immediately.

3 KNOW THYSELF

How did you end up in this condition? If you take a look at your history, you'll see that insomnia didn't just *happen* to you overnight. It was probably a while in the making, and you helped it along unknowingly with your lifestyle and mental care choices.

How Did You Get This Way?

Sleep deprivation due to increased consumption of sugar and stimulants like in energy drinks, soda and junk food, as well as not enough physical play and too much television / video game time, are now commonly acknowledged as contributing to ADHD in children. Today we prefer to pump children full of drugs if they seem a bit off to us, or if we need to settle them down--when a good number of these kids might just need a lot more time outside, a diet made of unprocessed food, and more sleep.

If you have children, you will remember how impossible your baby or toddler was with just *one* night of poor sleep, or even a missed nap. There is simply no hope of ease and harmony until the little one gets the right amount of sleep. How about your tween or teenager after a sleepover with friends? The next day is a complete write off. If they get a couple less hours of sleep than usual, they are no longer able to handle even simple responsibilities like grooming, chores, homework, manners.

As adults we manage our symptoms better, but it doesn't take much missed sleep to transform a balanced adult into that cranky, impossible toddler. Or worse. At the end of five years of severe insomnia, I had a huge, excruciatingly painful tumor in my liver, hypothyroidism, and arthritis. I could barely drive a car and I hated being alive. Now that I'm sleeping, all of these problems are gone.

You've probably heard it said that we are more sleep-deprived than we were in the past. It is said that we are sleeping nearly two hours less than we were forty years ago, when we were sleeping about 8.5 hours per night. There are many reasons for this. The main contributor is lifestyle changes due to electricity. Now most of us stay awake well after dark. Many people don't experience any separation between day and night. City dwellers are often totally removed from any connection to the cycles of the moon, and they have no idea which star is which. Most of us have never seen the swirls of the Milky Way.

Many people suffer from an inability to balance work and their personal lives as well. Modern work technology like tablets, phones and laptops makes it hard for us to ever be disconnected from work.. We have 24/7 internet, news, light, TV, so there is no "down" time. Without the natural down time, we sedate and self-medicate to slow down. Then we stimulate ourselves with ever higher doses of caffeine, even in younger and younger children, to keep up with the rush. Just in the last few years, I am frequently surprised and dismayed to find how many children as young as eleven I see with caffeinated or even decaffeinated (instead of caffeine-free) Starbucks' beverages! If you'd caffeinated me at that age, you'd have to peel my atoms off the ceiling! Now it's normal for tweens to drink caffeinated beverages regularly, and most high school kids are routinely caffeinated. It's a recipe for global mania and global insomnia.

It's also said that if it takes you more than fifteen minutes to fall asleep, you're sleep deprived. For insomniacs, sometimes it's a couple hours or more before you can sleep. Or you might be one of those people who don't fall asleep at all, all night long. Maybe you sleep two hours and then you're up the rest of the night, only to doze off right before you need to get up and go to work.

Insomniacs often feel like we can't shut off our brains. We feel trapped in our heads. Have you ever over-stimulated your infant, toddler or child and tried to put him or her to bed in fifteen minutes? Ain't gonna happen, no way. Sometimes it can take a couple hours to get an over-stimulated child to sleep. Sometimes when they're in this condition, they can't get into deep, relaxed sleep at all. They toss and turn all night long and everyone pays for it the next day with crabbiness and tantrums.

It's easier to see and manage sleep deprivation in children. We regulate every aspect of their lives much more strictly. We know if they don't sleep everyone suffers, especially them. We accept that their brains don't develop properly if they are under-slept. Where I live now, consultation with a sleep coach is part of regular post-natal care, funded by the government. When we change the clocks forward and back in spring and fall, experts have recommendations for how to prepare and transition your children through just this one hour change.

Adults are much less conscious and careful with ourselves. We push and push ourselves in so many ways, don't take any proper mental care, and then still expect to sleep, to shut off like a machine. It's not possible. Just because scientists haven't quite yet figured out all the reasons we need sleep doesn't mean we don't need it as much as we need food, water, and shelter. Our inability to understand the exact physiology and chemistry defining why we need sleep makes us much too casual about incurring sleep debt. (That's the cumulative effect of not getting enough sleep). Scientists still haven't agreed on how much sleep debt we can accumulate. But people will agree that when they were in their early twenties it was easier to pull an all-nighter than in their forties!

For the working mother, pressure can be particularly intense. You're expected, and you expect yourself, to be the successful breadwinner, efficient housekeeper, creative cook, loving mother, horny and sexy wife, educator, chauffeur, secretary; you still need time to bake cupcakes, garden so you can eat your own veggies, compost & recycle, spring clean and more and more and more.

Did you know that in the past to run a household the size of the modern suburban house, at least three indoor servants were required? Plus nanny, governess, gardeners, and workers to care for animals. Granted, today we have washers and dryers and cars. Nonetheless, if we are having a hard time juggling our personal lives and our careers we think something is wrong with us, that we're not working hard enough! How did that happen? For single parents, the stress gets over the top.

A single working mother's recreational, health and spiritual pursuits are the first to be sacrificed, even though pastimes such as exercise and meditation/prayer are fundamental to maintaining work/life balance. Often working mothers find themselves caught in this manic cycle with no break, day after day. We often expect ourselves to perform with robotic productivity levels & rest cycles. I know I do. It is an impossible situation and quickly makes us sick and exhausted with our families and our lives, and hard to live with.

And a bath before bed is supposed to sort you out?

What's the point of working so hard for your family if you're cranky and miserable all the time and your family members hate being near you?

Your Family History

Were you born a good self-soother? Or were you an angry, screaming baby? Some people are just light sleepers to start with, and people like this may develop insomnia more easily.

My husband trained in the Russian special forces. He has spent many nights sleeping in strange, uncomfortable, claustrophobia-inducing insecure places. Wearing too little clothing in the freezing cold. Wearing a full bio-hazard suit in the heat, sleeping in a tank with an inch clearance above his head. He now has the unique ability to sleep deeply anywhere, whether stretched out on an airport floor in Thailand, or on a cold train in Siberia. He doesn't need a pillow or the right mattress. He doesn't awaken until he's ready. He feels best with at least ten hours per night. If I go away somewhere with the kids for a weekend, he will take what I call a "sleeping holiday." This means that he spends the whole time sleeping. He just gets up occasionally to pee, eat a bit, watch a movie, take a short run, then back to sleep.

Not me. I'm high strung and very sensitive. Even now I only sleep well in my own bed with very particular blankets, no noise, no light, and a special bedtime meditation ritual. Snoring husband? Banished to the kids' bedroom. (That's why I bought my boys a double-sized bunk bed, so they can host their papa when he snores). I even wear construction headphones so I don't hear him snoring from there, or hear anyone get up to pee, or a car drive by, or a person talk from the street. Without the headphones, as soon as there's a creak of a bed anywhere in the house I'm awake. But that's not new. I've always been a light and low-volume sleeper. As a child, I was always the first one up. Frequently I'd awaken in the middle of the night too, but back then it didn't bother or tire me because I wasn't yet riddled with the anxieties of an adolescent or the cares of an adult. Back then it was fun to look around until I dozed off again.

Life progressed. I made some common but unfortunately self-sabotaging choices. I did a lot of all-nighters during university, fuelled by coffee. By my mid-twenties, I had Official Problems Sleeping. Any little noise would awaken me. I found it hard to get back to sleep. I'd get up and work, practice, write, caffeinate. Put my head down for a few minutes after lunch and drink more coffee. For the ten years I lived in San Francisco and Hollywood, I hardly had a single good night's sleep due to the relentless noise of inner city life.

Only during my years of severe insomnia did I research my family history. As it happens, no one on my mom's side of the family sleeps well. It seems to worsen with age in our family. My sister and brother both developed problems sleeping in their mid-thirties. My mother wakes frequently and easily. My dear uncle that I spoke of earlier may not have slept well for many, many years prior to my aunt's illness.

We now know that sleep-related behavior, such as when you want to sleep (morning person or night owl) and for how long you need to sleep, is regulated by genetics.[4] So if you come from a family of poor or light sleepers, you may inherit or develop this condition as you enter adulthood. Understanding your family history is very important. It will give you a good idea of what kind of goals to set for yourself. For example, for me, eight hours a night may not be possible. I'm not sure if I have ever slept for eight hours in a row. I mean, ever, in my lifetime. But with even six hours of good sleep, I feel like Superwoman. However, my husband wouldn't even last the day without a nap on six hours sleep per night.

One of my jobs required a lot of international travel, which messed up my internal clock and got me started with sleeping aids and over-caffeination. Even four Tylenol PMs wouldn't knock me out, but they left me in a terrible stupor the next day. I'd drink a pot of coffee, maybe more, and would emerge from the stupor mid-afternoon. Exercise after work gave me a jolt of energy to keep going. Then a couple evening martinis to wind down. It was during this time that I lost the habit of sleeping more than a couple hours at a time.

Sleep Cycles

From our perspective, sleep means we're "off", the same way you turn off a light. But in fact our minds are very busy at night. We have sleep cycles that are repeated through the night. We start in lighter sleep, move to deeper sleep, then to dream sleep, back to lighter sleep, then deep sleep, then dream sleep. We do this about five times a night, with each cycle being about ninety minutes. You have more deep sleep earlier on, and more dream sleep closer to the morning.

Child experts tell you that it's important to let babies learn to self-

---

[4] He Y., et al., "The Transcriptional Repressor DEC2 Regulates Sleep Length in Mammals," Science 325 (5942): 866-870. (2009)

soothe, otherwise each time they cycle up to lighter sleep, they'll wake up and expect you there to comfort them. These are the babies that cry every couple hours in the night. The babies who aren't natural self-soothers need to learn and practice the art of riding the sleep cycles on their own. Fortunately most babies learn pretty quickly, a lot faster than adults do once we've developed insomnia.

Grown-ups work pretty much the same way. Some of us are good self-soothers and can sleep right through the less-deep portion of our sleeping cycles (my husband). Some of us are poor self-soothers and wake up more easily (me). The poor self soothers are more quick to lose the habit of sleeping, but it doesn't happen overnight. When I look back, I see my trajectory laid out quite clearly. It took about six years to start sleeping only a couple hours at a time. Two hours sleep, two or three hours awake, busy with toxic thoughts of one kind or another, another hour and a half of sleep then bbzzzzzzzzzzz! Time to get up and get to work. Gimme dat coffee!

Sleeping is a Habit

Why do I call sleeping "a habit"? Because it's something you practice and get used to. That's what child experts tell us about our babies, and we're not so much different. Insomnia is also a habit; you practice being awake instead of asleep, and you get used to that. Your body does its best to help you out, shooting you full of stress hormones to keep you awake. To boot, mothers get some built-in hormonal boost to help them handle the sleep deprivation of newborn period.

Add that to the mix, and by the time I went home from the hospital with my firstborn, I was not even falling asleep for more than fifteen or thirty minutes at a time.

How do you train yourself to be an insomniac? Not only does it take a good chunk of your life, but we even work pretty hard at it: when we get up to work or watch television or exercise if we can't stay asleep. When we are not moderate in our intake—too much coffee, food, wine. When we commit to toxic thinking rather than right thought and right action. When we *prefer* toxic thinking to constructive problem solving. When we place really difficult expectations on ourselves, such as aggressive work schedules that require a lot of travel and / or shift work. As we do all these things, we train our bodies to sleep less deeply, to wake up more easily and more frequently, and to hunker down into survival mode so we can just keep rolling along.

It took me six years to lose the habit of sleeping more than a couple hours at a time, another five years of severe insomnia before I hit rock bottom and about only about three years to get back to healthy "normal" sleep habits—that's not such bad math!

The bottom line is that even if you've been sleeping poorly for years, you can still heal yourself a lot faster than it took you to get stuck in the insomnia abyss.

Isn't that great news?! I hope it inspires your patience and enthusiasm for this process. You must be patient, because you did this to yourself slowly. Possibly over many years, even decades. It's totally irrational to expect a quick-fix that doesn't involve your time and energy. Like a sleeping pill, for example. Not a single sleeping pill helps an insomniac sleep deeply all night long. Not a single one. You might start getting groggy, you might even sleep for a few hours. Then you wake up, take another, get groggy, maybe sleep a bit. Before you know it morning has come, and you don't even feel a bit rested, but you sure feel terrible. It takes you hours to get out of the chemical stupor; sometimes you don't get out of it until late afternoon. I tried a few sleeping aids--Tylenol PM, Ambien, Lunesta, and still didn't sleep, but drove a car and worked all day regardless of the hazy fog I was in. I needed so much coffee to function in this miserable substandard condition. Then vino and martinis for evening unwinding.

Not that they were helping anyway, but sleeping pills, coffee and alcohol were out of the question for the five years that I was pregnant and nursing, so I had self-medication to rely on, nothing to provide any false hope. I had to sort it out on my own or else. I'm grateful for this now, otherwise I may have clung to the fantasy that sleeping aids might have helped me.

Take a few moments to consider your own history:

- What kind of self-soother are you?
- How many years have you been sleeping poorly?
- What mix of circumstances and actions led up to it?
- Is your environment set up to accommodate you? For example, if you're a light sleeper, are you stuck beside someone who is snoring, or on a busy street? Are you still letting your kids crawl into bed in the middle of the night? Do you get to wake up naturally or are you woken up by others or an alarm?

- If you're in really bad condition now, what sent you over the edge? Shift work, family problem, health problem, work problem, PTSD?
- What crutches do you rely on? Drugs, food, stimulants, obsessions? For how long?
- How effective are they? How do you feel when you use them? Do you want to be free of them? Are you willing to do the work to be free of them?

We Worry A Lot About Not Sleeping

Paradoxically, much night-time anxiety for the insomniac focuses on whether we will sleep or not, and how we will manage if we don't. My normal, chaotic young children were so demanding and slept so poorly that I'd lie there and dread how I was going to get through the night, and then get through the day. Every day, for more than two years, I didn't know how I was going to survive the day. As the day waned, I began to worry if I'd sleep at all, and I felt I couldn't survive another night without sleep. Worry, fear, anxiety. This was very stressful and kept me from relaxing enough to fall asleep. So even if my kids were sleeping, I'd still be wide awake wondering how I was going to ever be well rested enough to take care of them.

How stupid is that? I knew exactly how stupid, and that's what made me get all stressed out about it in the middle of the night.

It's important to remind yourself that it took you years to get to this low. When you are training yourself to sleep again, you need to accept the fact that your recovery from this medical emergency is going to take some time. Why? Because very few of us are savants; most of us are experiential beings. This means we learn and understand and change only with practice, with repetition. In The Matrix movies, the humans can upload vast amounts of knowledge to their brains via computer circuitry which they can apply immediately, without practice. Need to be able to fly a helicopter in a war zone? Need to master multiple fighting styles? No problem; a five-second upload.

That's not the way it works for us in the real world. We need years and practice to master skills. Healing your trauma also takes practice. When you sprain your ankle, it's not miraculously healed overnight. You don't push yourself to run the next day. Maybe you get an x-ray to make sure nothing is broken; you use ice and elevate your leg. You don't walk or run or drive. Maybe you use a cane for a while; you go to physiotherapy and do exercises. Eventually you're able to run again, but not for a while.

After a heart attack, does the bypass patient get back to an aggressive schedule and fatty diet? No. Rehab and discipline are required to restore even normal functioning. Although the patient is impatient, s/he has no choice. That's what happens in a medical emergency. Your insomnia is also a medical emergency. You need to be patient as you readjust your life and practice new disciplines.

Even babies are mostly patient when learning to walk. Despite falling over and over, nothing can stop that baby from trying and practicing and trying and practicing. Deep inside that child, is the seed of success—he or she knows somewhere, somehow it's going to happen eventually; he or she has the instinct for faith. The baby's dogged determination and patience eventually pay off. Some kids learn sooner and some kids figure it out later, but most of them get there at some point. Same with you—sooner or later you'll get there. You must be patient with yourself and just keep trying. If even a baby, with incompletely developed brain function, can be patient and determined enough to pull it off, so can you. You need to shut off your mind chatter to make it happen.

Remember my very long list of problematic symptoms? These were the injuries I inflicted upon myself during my extended period of insomnia. You may have a similar or long list of new physical and mental problems. It took you a while to injure yourself in this way, training yourself to be an insomniac. Now you are committing to a lifestyle change. You want to teach yourself to sleep again, and if you are a good student it will be faster. That means paying attention, doing your homework, putting your heart and mind into it. If you don't follow through with practice, then it will take longer and maybe you won't get there.

The student doesn't expect to pass the class without putting in any work, and neither can you. The student knows patience and dedication are important. This means you must ride through sleepless periods with the best attitude you can. Your anxiety serves no purpose; it only slows you down by getting you into fight or flight mode in the middle of the night. The only thing you can do is practice gratitude. Gratitude is the panacea, the antidote for all nighttime toxic thinking, and it's a lot more effective than sleeping aids or anti-anxiety medications for calming your mind. For me it was so incredibly effective, its results so immediate, that I'm surprised scientists and doctors don't study and apply this technique, the same way the placebo effect is now used as a treatment in difficult-to-diagnose-and-treat cases.

Give Yourself What You Need

Once you've taken some time to understand your insomnia trajectory, don't fight or bemoan what's been. Don't blame yourself for getting into this rut. Don't blame others, either. Know thyself; know thy personality. Work with what you have. Why? Because in your fragile condition, you don't have the bandwidth to challenge your subconscious mind and expect big changes. If you are a light sleeper, you need quiet and no interruptions. Once you are sleeping again, then you can sleep with the snoring wife or someone who moves around in the bed a lot. But while you are in recovery, no way. Trying to change your nature at this point is not possible; it is asking too much of yourself. If you're a small town boy living next to the subway in a big noisy city, you are not going to be able to sleep well. It's time to consider moving or sound-proofing. Sound-proofing doesn't have to be expensive, either.

Some problems are not as easy to change, and you will need to understand those, too. If you are risk-averse but have surrounded yourself with instability, you won't sleep well. If you're stressed about something, you won't sleep well. You can't fix your insomnia if you don't take some action to solve the problems in life that are bothering you. There are a zillion maxims about this; they are all true! Right thought, right action, right relations, right livelihood—these make you a more peaceful sleeper. If your problems and the way you think about them have brought you to the point where you are unable to experience any delight and joy in day to day living, you need to make some changes to your thinking and to your actions. If you are just trying to take sleeping pills without making these changes, you are absolutely out of luck. There is no hope for sleep health down that path. Zero. You are pursuing an illusion, a complete fantasy.

A huge problem in my family is that my husband has bad drinking binges, didn't want to have kids in the first place, and resents their interference with his life plan and his freedom to explore and experiment. He never bothered to sort out a career path that he felt passionately about, and even now he despises working to make money to support our family. I love my husband's wild, undomesticated ways. I love that he is a strange wolf and thinks out of the box. If he wasn't I might not be attracted to him. But I was used to a very conservative and stable father, so after having kids I resented my husband enormously. I couldn't figure out what was wrong with him, that he didn't want to devote his life to our family like I was. For a new mother, the lack of support from your spouse is extremely stressful.

Russians are enormous drinkers, even the women, and my husband is no exception. He was basically drunk for the entire time I experienced severe insomnia. While perhaps normal for a Russian woman, for me this was crazy and insulting. Living with an addict is, well, terrible. I felt like the second wife, and Stolichnaya was the favorite one. One reason he was drinking so much was that it was stressful to be around me—I was paranoid, nervous, and angry, all the time. When I started sleeping more, he started drinking less. His drinking really stresses me out, so when he started drinking less I started sleeping just a little bit more.

To my husband's credit, he stood by me during those difficult years and is entirely responsible for researching and acquiring all the alternative natural cures we tried—the juicer for juice fasts, the Vita-Mix for blending superfood smoothies, an infrared sauna, yoga programs, a magnet-mattress, a grounding sheet, Chinese herbs, tonics & tinctures that he prepared himself, breathing masks, oxygen therapy, carbon dioxide therapy, fasting programs, growing wheatgrass and sprouts, buying a microscope powerful enough to view my bloodcells, a Gauss meter, a Geiger counter, fat calipers, a TDS water meter, EMF filters, and lots of other gadgets and meters for monitoring my bodily experiments. I would never have bothered with these things without his curiosity and efforts; I simply didn't have the energy and wherewithal for research and planning.

I'm editing this chapter while my youngest, now four, is zonked out on the sofa after having a Great Fit at the dentist's office. He got two caps and he was really mad about it. While I was driving us home, he undid his seatbelt and tried to jump out of the car. I managed to catch him by the hood of his coat, stuff him back in the car and race home. When we arrived he whacked me with a stick and ran down the block. My husband caught up with him, carried him for a few blocks until he calmed down, then bounced him on our trampoline for about thirty minutes until he fell asleep in his arms. So my husband's a good guy. (So is my son, but, man, does he have a temper!)

There were other stresses in my environment that contributed to my sleeping problems. In retrospect I know that I should have corrected these. But I just didn't know better at the time. When my first son was born, we were living in a tiny apartment in a big noisy city. I moved there from a giant, quiet house on the edge of a small city, where five minutes walk took me to farmers' hay fields and the largest urban park in North America. I was never peaceful or relaxed in inner city San Francisco or Los Angeles, but didn't realize this. I thought I'd be able to change my nature. I'm also a very high-strung person who gets anxious easily in high-risk situations. I don't like roller-coasters and zip lines and parachuting. I even vomit after a merry-go-round ride. Both professionally and personally, in my twenties I pushed myself into many irregular, stressful situations to "expand" my horizons but once again was trying to fight my nature, which requires variety but stability and peacefulness.

These kinds of stresses impact you subconsciously, and hence will impair the insomniac's attempts to restore sleep health. You need to make your environment and relations more comfortable. Often we don't even know what's bothering us. Some problems can be easily solved if we could but identify them. Often we're too busy just doing to stop and think, to ask and know. Take some time to understand what is making you tick and tock. Set your minimum standards and figure out how to communicate them respectfully and earnestly.

You must take actions to bring you some equilibrium regarding the problems that torment you, or you will not improve your sleep and you will get worse and sick. But even if you can't take action to solve the problem, you can change your thinking. Often this is even more powerful than action, as in the case of gratitude.

Shut out Judgment and Criticism

Many stresses that keep us up at night have to do with aspects of personal or professional relationships that are beyond our control. Here's where a change in thinking is required.

This is a hard pill to swallow for many people: you cannot control anything but your own mind. The actions and thoughts of others are not yours to control. Your attempts to do so can only lead to further misery and sleeplessness.

Conversely, the judgment and criticism of your family and colleagues can also keep you up at night. Here is another hard pill to swallow: their opinion of you is none of your business. You have a medical emergency to solve, and every neuron in your brain is needed.

An insomniac does not have one bit of energy to spare on the negative opinions of others.

Perhaps you think your circumstances are special and warrant nighttime worry, anger, and resentment. But you are not the only person that is bothered by the judgment and criticism of others. This is part of the human condition. Another fact of human nature that interferes greatly with sleep is our tendency to compare ourselves with others, either favorably or unfavorably. Frequently this is how we define our own worth and happiness.

Tied to this is our penchant for thinking the grass is greener somewhere else. We think that our problems are worse than somebody else's, or that our neighbor, boss, cousin, or that skinny stranger in the grocery check-out line, or the person driving that expensive car is happier and has an easier life.

Handling judgment and criticism is an inescapable part of being human. Nobody gets a pass. The best you can do is ride it with ease and grace. There is not a single person on the planet that garners enough respect or prestige to be above someone's criticism. Even Mother Teresa had critics.

Conversely, very few people have so much self-control that judging and criticizing others is beneath them, either. I've hung around some fairly enlightened folks who can't resist a dig at people they perceive to be pretentious.

Once again, you get to choose: do you want to be in control of the thoughts and actions of others, or do you want to learn to sleep again? Do you want to dedicate your thoughts and energy to useless and frustrating comparisons, or do you want to focus on your health and get your life back?

In a loving way, withdraw into your own bubble and shut out the noise that no longer serves your goal of sleep health. Comparing and judgment are thought patterns that no longer serve. Banish the thoughts, hundreds of times a day if you have to: *Begone, because this thought is none of my business and no longer serves me.* Then fill the hole with gratitude, because it makes happy hormones in your body, and these happy hormones pave the way to health: *I am grateful that I am dedicating my whole mind to my healing. I am grateful that I can make happy hormones just with my thoughts. Yes, yes, yes.*

You can't change your family or your colleagues, but you can certainly change your thinking about them. I was twisted up in knots for about year after my family blew me off when I hit rock bottom. In my mind it was a betrayal; I felt their love was shallow and conditional and lame.

If somebody I know has a problem, I'm one of those in-your-face friends, until it's fixed. In fact, I can be a pretty annoying busy-body and a preachy know-it-all. When I was in crisis, I expected my family to act like me, to pick up the pieces and figure it out, as I do for others. Even though others often dislike it when I do this! I judged them harshly because they weren't acting like me. I deemed them unworthy because they didn't make any room in their busy lives to help me sort out an enormous health mess that took me more than a decade to create. In other words, I was angry not because of their actions, but because I couldn't control their actions.

During my sleepless nights, these breakthroughs didn't come right away. In fact, it took about six months of Banish / Gratitude before I was able to direct my thoughts to forgiveness. I had to forgive them in order to forgive myself for being so controlling, arrogant and egocentric. For thinking that I was better than them, and that my way of doing things was the best way. That I could create a mess and expect others to clean it up.

Harvest the Wisdom

Once the light of forgiveness switched on, I was immediately able to hone in on the lessons to be learned from my time in crisis. Or, as they say, to harvest the wisdom. The lessons I learned are the key points of this book. You've seen them before, because they apply broadly to many of life's challenges:

- You alone are responsible for solving your problems. In this case, your problem is the medical emergency of insomnia.
- Your medical emergency will take some time, patience and discipline to solve. You need to want to heal more than you want anything else.
- You need mental care to solve this problem. It is your responsibility to give yourself mental care now and for the rest of your life.
- The foundation for mental care is quieting mind chatter and counting your blessings. This enables you to take right action.

My story provides an example of how you can change your thinking about a problem or issue. When you are able to change your thinking, it's a lot easier to leave the toxic thoughts behind. Some people learn fast, but not me: it took me five years in the insomnia abyss to figure out these basic life lessons.

What is the wisdom you can harvest from your problems? Take it. Seize it, focus on it, and practice leaving the rest behind with Banish / Gratitude.

Don't hesitate to seek out professional help to assist you in lining up right thought and right action. There's a lot of free or low-cost counseling that you can take advantage of if money is an issue. Even simply verbalizing what is bothering you in a constructive way, or writing down your thoughts in a journal often has the effect of giving you some distance from them. Jennifer Hadley uses a written exercise called The Forgiveness Letter, which is easy and effective (available for free at www.jenniferhadley.com) Once your problems are out of your head and on paper, they become more manageable. Stay focused on your goal and strategy: you are responsible for solving your medical emergency by restoring sleep health. You alone rule your mind.

Listen to Supportive Materials

Isn't it great to be alive the Age of Oprah Winfrey? I'm very grateful to be alive in a time and place where I won't get burned at the stake for thinking out of the box. There is such a wonderful supply of self-help material to assist you in choosing right thought and right action. Every library is packed full of multiple copies of Deepak Chopra, Esther Hicks/Abraham, Louise Hay, Marianne Williamson, Gary Renard, Wayne Dyer, David Hoffmeister, Doreen Virtue, and so on. The internet has even more free materials. There are thousands of videos on YouTube. Each of the gurus above has hours and hours of free audio classes and radio shows. The work of Jennifer Hadley has been very important in helping me change my thinking about my problems. She's easy to listen to, respectful of everyone's approach and the problems they present.

If you're up all night, I recommend that you listen to as many audio books and helpful materials as you can during this time. Many of the writers and teachers I cite above have meditation CDs and mp3 files. My favorite meditative listening materials were my own meditation albums, and material from wisdomcenter.com.

Why? If you're like how I was, you don't have the strength to keep your eyes open or hold up a book. My head and eyes usually ached too much for reading, but I disliked being awake listening to my mind-chatter, so listening to something else was the best option for me. I kept a night's worth of audio material on my old little MP3 player, and it often ran all night long. I kept it right next to me so that I could grab it and navigate through the files easily, without it causing me further agitation. Listening to this material is much more uplifting than your mind chatter and can help get you in a better mood. Try to relax and just enjoy being awake and listening. Since you're going to be awake anyway, don't fight it; that only produces the stress hormones that get your heart racing and make you heat up. Plus you can learn a lot, and when you're listening all the time, every night, the thoughts sink in and come back to you easily during the day. Also, if you relax and listen to interesting books, programs and classes, you are likely to doze off, since you stop making stress hormones when you aren't dwelling on your problems.

Below is some of the material I found most helpful. I listened to all of it, rather than reading it, and most of it during the nights I was awake:

The books of Abraham, written by Esther Hicks, about the Law of Attraction. Essentially Abraham's point is that the purpose of our life is to be happy, in every moment, and we can easily follow our emotions as a guide. They have a daily thought you can get in email from Abraham-Hicks.com; it's a nice meditation for starting the day, a reminder of what your priorities should be and how you should direct your thoughts in positive, loving directions. There are also many written exercises for helping you figure out right action to get from where you are to where you want to be.

Brian Tracy, a famous selp-help guru, talks about unconditional forgiveness of everyone all the time—yourself, parents, family & others— as the mark that distinguishes a successful, happy person from one who is "stuck." When I find myself clinging to anger, blaming someone else in the middle of the night, I hear his voice in my head saying "you must forgive everyone of everything all the time. Not just 70 times 7!" He doesn't sugar coat anything.

Deepak Chopra. What can I say? Despite his decades of fame, I'd never read or listened to any of his work until my time in the insomnia abyss. My mom talked about him a lot when I was younger, and I used to roll my eyes. But I have since found that every single publication is so incredibly helpful for developing mindfulness practice in a way that makes sense to Westerners. It's also masculine and concrete, and easier for men to listen to than perhaps some other self-help work, which is too emotionally oriented.

Doreen Virtue (DoreenVirtueLLC.com) is a counselor whose take on life is so loving that it is a pleasure to immerse oneself in her world. She has numerous books, classes, and a weekly radio show at hayhouseradio.com

The work of Gregg Easterbrook in the <u>Progress Paradox</u> has been really helpful for me in understanding that depression, unusually high expectations, and unusually low tolerance for life's necessary "downs" is part of the modern malaise.

Eventually I was led to <u>A Course in Miracles</u>, which is a non-denominational spiritual text. In fact, it was life changing for me. If I had to pick one book to be marooned with on a desert island, this would be the book. Jennifer Hadley (www.jenniferhadley.com), Gary Renard, Marianne Williamson, Ronda Britten and David Hoffmeister are also excellent teachers of the course whose books I have listened to. In a nutshell, the Course teaches that human suffering is rooted in judgment of one's self and others, and it is our job to give love and be happy by practicing forgiveness through the releasing of judgment and expectation. Big words. Lots of change in thinking required for us mere humans to accomplish, but the rewards are immediate and enormous. If you're a person who's ever had a hankering to understand what it's all about, what your life purpose is, and other metaphysical / epistemological questions, you will be delighted by this book. If you're familiar with the Course, you will by now recognize that it informs my thoughts about fixing your insomnia.

There is no need to listen to a lot of audio books to teach yourself to sleep. However; this is a more fun, relaxing and helpful way to pass the time if you're awake at night. Every one of these writers and thinkers advocate a mental practice that requires discipline to achieve; that's the important part. If you're used to holding a grudge, it might take some time to develop the willingness to let go of your resentment. Listening to helpful material can assist you to develop the willingness, and is easier to listen to than your own thoughts.

Remember, when you are not willing to let go, it means you value the grudge and what it gives you more than you value what sleep can give you.

The Rewards of Getting Into Mental Shape

If you are stubborn and thick like me, you might need to do

banish-gratitude for months about a single issue. But just like getting in physical shape, getting into "mental" shape has massive rewards:

- It will help you fall back asleep when you awaken.
- It will help you stay asleep for longer.
- It will help you stay relaxed when you are awake at night.
- It will help you handle the exhausting hard days with more hope, ease and grace.

And, it will accomplish the above in less time than it took you to unconsciously create your sleeping problem in the first place. Why? Remember that powerful, multi-billion dollar tool you have? It's called intention. Once your conscious *intention to heal* is in the game—in this case your intention to restore healthy sleep—you can accomplish a lot in less time. Just try it and see.

At the very least it's better than lying awake angry and fearful. You have nothing to lose and everything to gain.

Summary

- It took you a while to become an insomniac. Take some time to understand the trajectory that led you to this point. Frequently, our lifestyles and choices over many years have promoted poor sleep health.
- Learning about your family's history of sleeping problems can help you set realistic goals for yourself.
- Be patient; it will take some time to fix yourself. The good news is that if you're committed, it won't take as long to fix yourself as it took you to become an insomniac.
- Sleep is a habit you can practice or break. Just as babies need to be trained to self-soothe during the sleep cycles at night, we need to train ourselves to sleep again once we've broken the habit.
- Know your preferences and your personality and don't fight them. Take necessary action to accommodate your needs or you'll be bothered at night.
- Shut out the opinions and judgments of others and focus your thoughts and energy on your important goal of restoring sleep health.
- Support and amplify your efforts by reading and listening to positive self-help material, to help you shut out useless night-time mind chatter.

4 THE MYSTERY BEHIND YOUR NON-SLEEPING BODY

Once my kids were sleeping at least four hours in a row most nights, imagine my surprise to discover that I *still* couldn't sleep, at all! I locked myself in the basement. Spent the night at my mom's or a friend's house. I'd do all the right things—yoga and meditate before bed, nice bath, warm sleepy-time tea, but still lie there awake, all night, heart racing. Here was my one chance to get a good night's sleep. All I needed was a good night's sleep. There's nothing sleep can't fix. I knew it, down to the bone. And I'd blow my chance, night after night. I had no idea why, but it sure made me upset. I couldn't even accomplish something that simple and important as a good night's sleep. How was I going to raise kids, make a living? The only thing in my way was me. Not kids, not snoring, not street noise, not coffee, not anger at my family or husband, nothing. Only incomprehensible, defective me. Loser.

What the Heck is Wrong with My Body and Brain?

I tried my best to stay calm, but deep down I felt betrayed by my own body for being so out of my own control. I was hopping mad about it, and that made it even harder to sleep, of course.

I spent about five years sleeping only a handful of consecutive hours each week. How did I go on so long in this condition?

My local newspaper recently covered the story of an injured suburban hare. For more than three weeks, city wildlife officials received reports from residents who'd spotted the hare with an arrow pierced right through its abdomen, coming out the back. There's a happy ending: eventually the officials trapped and treated the poor bunny, who by now is recovered from its severe injuries and released back to the wild. Like this animal, I have no idea how I made it through the years of crisis. How did this bunny avoid bleeding to death? Or dying of pain, shock, gangrene or any of the other problems that can arise when you are running about with an arrow through your body?

Like that bunny, I'm very grateful to have survived. Now that I'm recovered, I can't imagine being back in that abyss. I don't think I could survive it again, honestly, but who knows? Humans, like pigs and rats and cockroaches, are pretty durable organisms. Even if we get a little sleep, we can do minimum self-repair, enough to keep slogging on.

I've tried every conventional solution and found them totally ineffective to somewhat helpful, from sleeping vacations to sleeping clinics; hypnotherapy, melatonin, and valerian, and so on. I was not a passive insomniac by any means. So why was it so hard to find an answer? Why did this stuff seem to work for other people but not for me? What was wrong with me? Why was my hardware so defective? Was I stuck this way forever?

Nothing is Wrong That Chemistry Can't Fix

I dreaded the third day after not sleeping two nights. On the third day I fell apart. My normal personality was gone. I was vicious, angry, nasty. Tantrums, shaking, vertigo, despair; suicidal and violent thoughts; in a blind rage at everyone around me. There was no joy and everything seemed black. I knew I shouldn't dwell on the problems that bothered me, but I couldn't seem to help it. The only thing that gave me energy was anger. I stumbled around in a black haze, too tired to walk up the stairs but dragging myself up them; too tired to drive but doing it anyway, physically incapable of stuffing my kids into their car seats. It sometimes took ten minutes to complete this task because I'd have to stop and rest in between kids or I'd faint. I'd just let one jump around the car while the other one screamed bloody murder in his seat. When I was ready I'd get up and try to get my oldest in the car seat.

The paranoia and rage were the worst. I felt so angry all the time, at my inner circle and at total strangers. I felt everyone was out to get me, laughing at me, filled with *schaddenfreude,* enjoying my misery.

Usually on the third night I'd get a couple hours sleep in a row, and the rage and paranoia disappeared. Then the cycle started again, and I was back to the third day disaster. It was only when I started sleeping a few hours in a row every day that I realized the anger, rage and despair were connected to the sleeplessness. Even on just a couple hours of sleep per night, I was capable of experiencing joy in routine activities. If I didn't sleep, mere existence filled me with rage and despair.

The immediacy of this connection between my mood and my sleep made me suspect a chemical issue was involved. Before this time, I felt that psychological issues alone were responsible for the sleeplessness. I'd only studied biology briefly in junior high school (that's middle school for Americans), and didn't know a thing about body chemistry. The realization that a chemical problem was at play was very liberating for me. Chemical problems can be solved more rationally than psychological problems, which are so nebulous and usually require a lot more time and effort to sort out.

It was also the first time I realized my post-partum depression was caused by sleeplessness instead of the other way around. The hormone balancing act you perform after having a baby is a lot harder without sleep. As soon as I was sleeping just a little bit, I wasn't feeling depressed at all. Many of my most severe symptoms of post-partum depression were actually the results of sleep deprivation, including the depression itself. I don't think this is something the medical system understands. It's known that many depressed adults suffer from sleep loss—as far back as 1993 a study concluded about 90%.[5] However, I believe it is the sleep loss itself that contributes significantly to the depression. In my experience, this was definitely the case.

There's a reason people say sleep on it and you'll feel better! In this chapter I will explain why, from a chemical perspective. Scientists now understand that insomnia is a physiological state of hyper-arousal. Blood pressure, heart rate, brain metabolic activity and stress hormones are higher. My sense that I was never "quite off" was exactly right, from a hormonal and chemical perspective: insomniacs don't shut down the way healthy sleepers do.

---

[5] Mann, Joseph John and David J. Kupfer, Biology of Depressive Disorders: Subtypes of Depression and Comorbid Disorders, Part 2 (Google Books, 1993).

Why Sleeping Pills Don't Help You Sleep

Instead of recognizing my medical emergency and taking appropriate action, I was preoccupied with guilt about my negativity and narcissism. I felt I should have been experiencing only motherly joy, no matter how tired I was.

I believe my uncle's severe chronic insomnia was also a cause of his depression and eventual psychosis. He didn't have the tools and discourse at his disposal that I did to sort himself out on his own. The medical system did nothing to help him. In fact, their negligence killed him. Pharmaceuticals weren't helping him sleep. He frequently stated he didn't sleep at all. Part of this might be due to sleep misperception--this is when you think you are not sleeping, but you are actually in light sleep. What is true is that you are not getting much restful deep sleep or dream sleep, the two states that are critical to self-healing.

The big question is, why were sleeping pills not helping him sleep? What's wrong with sleeping pills? Why do we bother with sleeping pills when they have no capability to help us fix insomnia? One reason we continue to rely on sleeping pills is ignorance. People don't understand how the chemistry works, hence they never realize why the pills can't address sleeping problems. They also don't understand the risks involved! If they did, they would think twice before starting the habit. Another reason for this dependency is the modern culture of pharmaceutical overuse. Big pharmaceutical companies have carefully fostered this culture with lavish, targeted spending over decades. Their sole aim is to make a bigger profit at the expense of naïve, tired humans.

The most common sleeping pills we use today are nonbenzodiazepines. These are thought to be "safer" than benzodiazepines (like valium) since they have less risk of overdose. However, the rest of the side effects are the same so the "non" is misleading to the layperson. Although the drugs have different chemical structures, they work identically—they enhance one of our neurotransmitter effects that promotes relaxation (benzodiazepines enhance the effect of the neurotransmitter gamma-aminobutyric acid, or commonly known as GABA, at the GABA receptor). Some of the effects are sedative, (less excitement), hypnotic (sleep inducers), anxiolytic (anti-anxiety), anti-convulsants and muscle relaxants.

Neither type of drug was meant to be used long term because

- They create tolerance (you get used to them and require a higher dosage to create the same effect),

- They create dependence (addiction), and
- They cause a difficult withdrawal syndrome when you try to get off them. For example, one symptom of the withdrawal is…insomnia!

The elderly are more prone to long term negative side effects as well as more serious side effects. One frustrating symptom of withdrawal is called rebound insomnia. This is when the insomnia caused by withdrawal from the drug is actually worse than your original insomnia. Panic attacks and depression are also part of the withdrawal syndrome. Other side effects include increased cancer risk, liver problems, and depression. Studies find that long term users of sedative hypnotic drugs (drugs that calm you down & induce sleep) have a higher risk for suicide and increased risk of death![6] Women don't metabolize the drugs as quickly as men do, and are more likely to spend the next day in a stupor and develop liver problems. The liver problems arise because your liver can't actually get the drugs out of your body. If you're not sleeping well, your organs aren't doing their best work anyway, so it's that much harder for you to clean the gunk out.

So, why aren't these pills helping me sleep? Because they are not chemically designed to help you sleep and restore healthy sleep habits. They are just not capable of it. They are not intended for it. A sleeping pill is merely a crude chemical slingshot, riddled with so many sleeping limitations it is surprising we even bothered to coin the term "sleeping pill." That is a complete misnomer. We think if we take a pill we'll zonk out and feel rested the next day. That's what we want. This is a complete fantasy. This pill does not exist. We repeat the same fantasy every day, popping the pills before bed, popping another in the middle of the night. Day after day, we cling to this fantasy despite mountains of personal experience telling us that it's not working like we want it to.

Sleeping pills might shorten the time it takes you to fall asleep, and they might reduce alertness during the night, but they worsen sleep quality by increasing your lighter sleep and decreasing deep sleep.[7]

---

[6] Kripke, D.F., "Greater incidence of depression with hypnotic use than with placebo," BMC Psychiatry 7:42(Aug 21, 2007).
[7] Maiuro, Roland D., Handbook of Integrative Clinical Psychology, Psychiatry, and Behaviorial Medicine: Perspectives, Practices and Research (Springer Publishing Company, 2009) 128-130. Also, Buscemi N., et al, "Manifestations

That's what's happening when you take a sleeping pill and you feel loopy without feeling sleepy: you're not reaching deep sleep. In fact, sleeping pills actually *hinder your ability* to reach the critical, restorative sleep state called slow-wave sleep. In addition, the rebound insomnia is often accompanied with agitation and anxiety. The longer-acting drugs have residual effects on your chemistry, and accumulate in your liver. That's the fog you feel all through the next day. The shorter-acting drugs which you process faster have more severe withdrawal symptoms (insomnia, agitation, depression for starters).

Are these negative side effects enough to turn you off of pharmaceutical sleeping aids?

The bottom line is this: when you take sleeping pills, you are creating a new and big health problem to manage, on top of your old one, insomnia. And to boot, you are creating worse insomnia. At no point are you are going to improve your sleep. So if you're thinking about getting a sleep aid, don't. If your doctor recommends it, rip up the prescription. If you're already on them, get the help you need to get weaned off. They have zero benefit in restoring your healthy sleep habits, and they inflict a lot of harm.

You are better off staying awake at night than taking sleeping pills. The improvements you can make to your sleeping through behavioral adjustments are much more effective and have no side effects. In truth, the only reason that sleeping aids have cornered so much of the insomnia market is because of human nature: as usual, we want an easy answer to a bad problem we made. We want an instant answer to a problem it took us quite a while to manifest. We don't want to have to think or work or do anything; we just want insomnia gone. We don't want to focus our intention to our own health because we are used to wasting it on criticism and self-criticism. We don't have any energy reserves for thinking or working or fixing. We are too exhausted; we are outwitted, broken. We want to believe the lie, that private companies want to help us feel better, as well as make their money. Nothing wrong with that. We don't want to believe they'd do something bad to us or mislead us. Because people who do bad things and cheat get stopped by the law, right? Wrong. Big companies use their money to tap-dance their way around the ethics that the rest of us had to learn in kindergarten. Stay away from sleeping pills.

---

and Management of Chronic Insomnia in Adults: Summary, Evidence Report and Technology Assessment, Number 125 (Agency for Healthcare Research and Quality, June 2005).

Barbiturates are the other type of drug that has been used as a sleeping aid. It's too easy to overdose on barbiturates (think Judy Garland, Marilyn Monroe, Jimi Hendrix) so they are no longer prescribed as sleeping aids and anti-anxiety medications. But they are still used for anesthesia, physician assisted suicide and lethal injection. The way they interact with your brain is even more potent and unstable. Barbiturates potentiate the same GABA receptor while also inhibiting (or depressing) the principal excitatory neurotransmitter in our brain (AMPA receptors). Basically you take a bit too much and over-relax your muscles so that you stop breathing. Luminal (phenobarbitol) is the most common barbiturate we hear of today.

When you read how these drugs work, it seems shocking that we would take such a risk with our bodies and minds. Our culture's "war against drugs" leads us to believe that prescription drugs are "safer" than illegal street drugs but once you explore how the chemistry works, you see that the pharmaceuticals are dangerous, too. Fortunately, I never developed a physical or psychological dependence on sleeping aids. If you have an addiction or tolerance for these, you will have to solve your insomnia plus the withdrawal syndrome, which will be worse than the insomnia you starting with in the first place! You may need professional help for this. It is worth it, because the sleeping pills simply can't help you restore permanent sleep health. They are a complete waste of your time, money and, most importantly, your hope.

You Can Fix Your Chemical Problem

Once I'd gotten it through my thick skull that I had a chemical problem, and not just a psychological problem, I got to work. Chemical problems were something I could figure out how to control and fix. How? With a plan, some experiments, time, and a way to track results. My husband loves this kind of stuff, so he jumped on board right away. Once I was sleeping a bit every day I was able to handle this kind of left-brained thinking. I could have never engaged in such sequential, forward-thinking activity when sleeping every third day. It was the practice of Banish / Gratitude that got me to sleep a few hours in a row every day.

At this point I had the brain capacity and energy to do some research about the chemical components of insomnia. Now I was able to loosely hypothesize about my condition. I was able to experiment upon myself and write down what happened and how I felt. I adjusted the variables and tracked those, too, and compared everything. Even just a little sleep pulled me out of the foggy pit of despair, and back into the busy world.

I learned that our body's chemistry plays a huge role in helping us sleep and also in keeping us awake when we should be asleep. Some medical professionals reading this might be tempted to dismiss my layperson's shallow understanding of this complex field. No offense, but you can kiss my ass, since you are part of the same medical establishment that helped my uncle die. These pages here contain what worked for me, the summary of a few years of self-experimentation and research, and I try to write in a way that is easy to understand. When I was in the insomnia abyss, I didn't have the ability to digest, interpret and retain technical reading material, and I keep that in mind for my own writing.

I didn't have access to the science journals where most of the research on sleeping is published, so it actually took me a while to find web-based information about sleep and body chemistry / hormones. Today, there's much more information on this topic available in the public arena than even just a few years ago. Wonderful Wikipedia is my first stop for all questions, and the detailed footnotes in each article are a godsend. But when I was in the abyss, between 2008-2010, it was harder to find information. My first gold nugget was an obscure study from an East Asian holistic institute. I've since lost the reference or I'd credit them here; their ideas were very insightful for me. I hope that Western general practice medicine will soon connect the insomnia and hormone dots that now seem so obvious to me, having lived through it. When you go to your doctor for help sleeping, they need to talk to you first about how to change your body chemistry on your own, instead of just giving you a prescription for sleeping aids, anti-anxiety medication or anti-depressant medication.

For the sake of non-technical clarity, I group hormones, enzymes, and neurotransmitters into a group I call "chemicals." A hormone is a chemical released by one part of the body that affects the whole body. A neurotransmitter is a chemical released by nerve cells in the brain and used to communicate with other nerve cells. An enzyme is a molecule that is responsible for the chemical reactions in our body that sustain life. They help change something into something else. They help us change our food into the hormones and neurotransmitters we need. We don't make any bad chemicals. Each one has its necessary purpose. It's more a matter of timing, quantity and balance. Good thing is that with the right food, the right thoughts, some exercise, we can usually get these parameters right!

The Insomniac's Chemical Problem

The chemical problem faced by the insomniac works like this: when you're chronically sleep deprived:

- Your body doesn't get the repair time necessary to make and use helpful chemicals, and to get rid of stress hormones,
- Your body makes stress hormones at inappropriate times,
- Your body doesn't make enough of the helpful chemicals or use them in the way that is most beneficial to you:

    1. Melatonin (makes us sleepy)
    2. Testosterone (helps men lower stress)
    3. Oxytocin (helps women lower stress)
    4. Serotonin (the "feel good" neurotransmitter for men and women
    5. Dopamine (the neurotransmitter that keeps us motivated, enthusiastic)

I approached the psychological component of my insomnia by making some lifestyle changes, particularly by developing a rigorous practice of mindfulness, where I directed my attention away from anger and other toxic thoughts. But this still didn't fix the chemical problem that kept me awake with a racing heart. I could be relaxed regardless at night, but still not able to fall asleep!

Our bodies have an internal clock for making stress chemicals, helpful chemicals, and well as melatonin (that's our sleeping hormone). When you're an insomniac, you and the clock don't sync up well. You also disable production capacity, so you don't make enough of the good stuff. Our helpful chemicals help us sleep, de-stress, and are connected to the self-healing capacity of our body. Not only do they help you make melatonin, the hormone that makes you sleepy, but they also help you make the other miraculous self-healing internal medicines we need to run optimally, like the lymph juice that keeps your teeth and gums strong, as well as interleukins, your very own potent anti-cancer medicine.

Even from this quick summary you can easily see how the vicious cycle sucks more and more of your body into its swath of destruction.

The lack of sleep compromises your body's ability to clean and repair itself, so that it becomes harder and harder to process your stress hormones and make happy chemicals. You start sleeping even more poorly. Your organs don't work as well since they don't get the needed down-time for repair. The outcome? You are packed with stress hormones and toxins that you can't get rid of efficiently, completely or easily. So you feel terrible and start sleeping even more poorly. You might have a harder time digesting food, absorbing nutrients, and pooping, and then you feel that much worse, so your sleep gets even worse. Down and down you go.

The result of your body's laboratory can be summed up as follows:

__The less you sleep, the more you lose the ability to sleep.__
__The more you sleep, the more you restore the ability to sleep.__

Sleep 101

Some animals can go without sleep for a long time, like baby killer whales and some dolphins, who don't sleep for the first month of their lives. But most mammal babies sleep for a good portion of the 24-hour day to help grow their brains and bodies. Even hibernating animals, though they wake up well-rested, immediately go into what's known as rebound sleep which they didn't get while hibernating. Some marine mammals sleep one cerebral hemisphere at a time so they can stay on the move even while they are sleeping. Some humans have set amazing records for the number of days without sleep. Some people are born with a gene that makes them need less sleep (DEC2). But most of us adults need to sleep about seven hours a night, and most of us feel better with a bit more.

For children it's a lot more sleep. Nine to ten hours for teenagers, eleven to twelve for younger children, and twelve to eighteen more for babies. We are careful about regulating total sleep time for our small children. But the digital age has quickly reduced the number of hours that teenagers sleep. I know some teenagers who play video games until midnight even though they need to start their day at six o'clock in the morning. Then, of course, they are crabby and feel terrible. They are unkind to their parents and siblings. They are filled with negativity and resentment. They can't focus in school. Normal teenage ups and downs are exacerbated with some of the personality changes caused by sleep deprivation, such as increased resentment, and a sense of victimization and a sense of self-entitlement. Then teens caffeinate at Starbucks at lunch time, stay up late again, and repeat. I expect we will need to direct significant thought as to how to make teens pay better mind to their sleep health, because the mental health implications are concerning.

You literally fall apart without sleep. This is a limitation of human mechanics. For a growing body it's that much more crucial. The myriad of intricately complex systems that keep us ticking, that we take for granted, grows more and compromised. One by one these systems just stop working well. Some of these systems do their best or only work at night. That's why the insomniac develops serious health problems quickly. For example, sleep is known as an anabolic state, which means we do our growing and generating during sleep. Slow-wave sleep, or "deep sleep" (NREM-3) is when we make growth hormone. Men who get less deep sleep have been make a lot less growth hormone[8], which is very important to keeping men healthy and manly. It's pretty important to women, also. Growth hormone not only determines your size but also your longevity; it's what promotes cell regeneration. We age prematurely without enough growth hormone.

Recent studies on mice by Dr. Allan Pack at the Center for Sleep and Circadian Neurobiology at the Perelman School of Medicine at the University of Pennsylvania show that a biological function called protein-folding, which is a critical part of cell growth and repair, is derailed.[9] Our cells, when sleep-deprived, are stressed out, and they can't do their jobs properly.

The memory and other cognitive problems I reported? I still can't speak my non-native languages very well anymore, and I find it extremely difficult to memorize piano repertoire now. I used to memorize pieces within a few a times of playing them well, without even trying to remember them; the notes were just there, in my fingers. I'm hoping this will be restored with time but so far haven't had any improvement. There are plenty of studies that show how sleep loss affects all sorts of cognitive functions—your memory, your ability to learn, your decision-making ability, your reasoning ability and more.[10] It's during sleep that knowledge and experience /

[8] Van Cauter, E et al, "Age-related changes in slow-wave sleep and REM sleep and relationship with growth hormone and cortisol levels in healthy men," Journal of the American Medical Association 284(7): 861-868 (2000).
[9] Cited by Luiza Ch. Savage, "The Sleep Crisis," Maclean's (June 24, 2013), 50.

memories get solidified and organized.[11] We make new neuron connections at night when we're sleeping. We have to do it then, because the physical way we accomplish this job doesn't allow for multi-tasking. While our while our body is doing this important work, we can't take in any external information.[i] So that's why it happens when we're asleep.

And that's why if you don't sleep enough or deeply, then you will see the problems manifest quickly. There have been tests done on some rats that showed their immune systems are suppressed as much as 20% from just short-term sleep deprivation[12], and their wounds heal more slowly.[13] Some poor rats that were kept awake indefinitely developed skin lesions, compulsive eating issues, loss of body mass, hypothermia and eventually fatal sepsis.[14] Lovely.

We don't actually need to kill rats to know what happens to people without sleep. There happens to be an extremely rare condition called Fatal Familial Insomnia, a brain disease without known cure caused by an inherited genetic mutation. The average survival span for patients with the onset of symptoms is only eighteen

[10] There are numerous articles citing these results. Some include Turner, T.H. et al, "Effects of 42 hour sleep deprivation on component processes of verbal working memory," Neuropsychology 21(6): 787-795 (2007); Daltrozzo et al, "Working Memory is Partially Preserved During Sleep," PLoS One 7(12) 2012; Born, J. et al, "Sleep to Remember," Neuroscientist 12410 (2006); Datta, S, "Avoidance task training potentiates phasic pontine-wave density in the rat: A mechanism for sleep-dependent plasticity," The Journal of Neuroscience 20 (22): 8607-8613 (2000); Kudrimoti, H.S, et al, "Reactivation of the hippocampal cell assemblies: Effects of the behavioral state, experience and EEG dynamics," The Journal of Neuroscience 19(10) 4090-4101 (1999); Marshall et al, "The Role of Sleep in Cognition and Emotion," Annals of the New York Academy of Sciences (1156:174 (2006).
[11] Stickgold, Robert, "Sleep dependent memory consolidation," Nature 437 (7063): 1272-8 (2005).
[12] Zager, A, et al, "Effects of acute and chronic sleep loss on immune modulation of rats," Regulatory, Integrative and Comparative Physiology 293: R504-R509 (2007).
[13] Gumustekin, K., et al, "Effects of sleep deprivation, nicotine, and selenium on wound healing in rats," International Journal of Neuroscience 114(11): 1433-42 (2004).
[14] Institute for Laboratory Animal Research, "Sleep deprivation of over 7 days with the disk over water system results in the development of ulcerative skin lesions, hyperphagia, loss of body mass, hypothermia and eventual septicemia and death in rats," Guidelines for the Care and Use of Mammals in Neuroscience and Behavioral Research, 121.

months. For the first four months, the patient has worsening insomnia, resulting in panic attacks, paranoia and phobias. For the next few months the patient experiences more hallucinations and severe panic attacks. The complete inability to sleep comes next, and after this rapid weight loss. This lasts for about three months and is followed by dementia, where the patient is unresponsive, and eventually dies. The most well known case of this disease is a Chicago music teacher who lived only six months after the onset of symptoms. (Don't panic; there were only eight diagnoses of this problem worldwide by July 2005, so it is extremely rare.)

Your Internal Clock

Insomniacs are generally not well aligned with our internal clocks. All living things on earth have such an internal clock, also called a circadian rhythm. This includes everything from bacteria and birds to hibernating animals and plants and people. In people, light plays an important role in setting our clock. There is plenty of individuation: we've got "morning" people and "night owls"—but even so, their natural wake and sleep times only vary by a couple or few hours. Our circadian rhythm influences sleep, body temperature, blood pressure, production of hormones and digestive secretions and more. This clock is actually a part of our brain (*suprachiasmatic nucleus*)—in the hypothalamus above where the optic nerves cross. (That's why it's sensitive to light.) Your sleep cycles are also influenced by your internal clock. During the day you've been making adenosine, a neurotransmitter that inhibits many of the body processes associated with wakefulness. Your internal clock tells your brain it's time to sleep and the chemicals you've made to start winding down kick in: about 9pm your body starts secreting melatonin, your sleeping hormone, and you start thinking about going to bed.

Eventually you get there, you lie down and relax. Your body temperature and blood pressure drop. You nod off. Your brain waves go from beta (active state) to alpha (relaxed state) as you descend into your first, drowsy sleep (NREM-1). You fall asleep and descend to NREM-2. Your brain makes theta waves and it's harder to awaken you. You've stopped twitching and jerking. Then you enter NREM-3, or deep sleep. Your brain makes delta waves; this stage is also called slow-wave sleep. Adenosine builds up in your brain. More chemicals get to work—acetylcholine secretion induces REM sleep, where most of your dreaming happens.

The Sleep Cycle (about 90 minutes)

- **Stage NREM1** (Non-Rapid Eye Movement). Brain activity consists of beta waves (that's "awake" brain waves) transitioning to alpha waves. This is your first stage between sleep and wakefulness.
- **Stage NREM2** comes next. Brain activity consists of theta waves and it's harder to wake you up.
- **Stage NREM3** is your deepest sleep, sometimes called "slow-wave sleep." Your brain emits delta waves. You are hardest to awaken in this stage, and you get more of this kind of sleep earlier in the night (during the first two sleep cycles).
- **REM Sleep** (Rapid Eye Movement) is when most dreaming happens. You're hard to awaken, and you have limp muscles (atonia or paralysis). You make lots of different kinds of brain waves--alpha, beta ("awake") and desynchronous waves. You get more REM sleep in the cycles closer to waking.

One of the most pervasive misconceptions about sleep is that sleep is just a matter of our bodies "turning off" for several hours, followed by our bodies "turning back on" when we awake. Most of us think of sleep as a passive and relatively constant and unchanging process. In fact, sleep is a very active state. Our bodies move frequently, as we roll about during the night, and our brain activity is even more varied than it is during the normal waking state, especially while we're dreaming. We're not "off" at all while we're sleeping; we're very busy doing very important stuff to keep ourselves healthy and sane.

This sleep cycle takes about 90 minutes, and you repeat it 4 or 5 times during the night, with more deep sleep (NREM 3) earlier in the night, and more REM (dreaming) later in the night. Your internal clock wants to drop your cortisol levels to coincide with your deepest sleep, between midnight and 2am, or about three hours after you go to bed. Your lowest body temperature naturally happens about 4:30am. Your body makes melatonin, grows bones, heals injuries, and engages in all sorts of miracles. We don't know exactly why we dream, but scientists know that REM sleep is very important to certain types of memory, so dreaming is important and necessary. Yet many insomniacs will tell you it's been years since they felt they last had a dream.

Closer to waking you get a rise in cortisol, a stress hormone secreted by the adrenal glands. This is called the cortisol awakening response. It's thought that this is to help us get organized to face the anticipated activities of the day quickly, our own natural morning cup of joe. It is said that how much you secrete is largely genetically determined—for example, "morning people" make more—and it's also influenced significantly by stress. You make more on a workday, and less when you have a day off.

Your Internal Body Clock - the Circadian Rhythm

2:00am - Deepest sleep
4:30am - Lowest body temperature
6:45am - Sharpest rise in blood pressure
7:30am - Melatonin secretion stops
8:30am - Bowel movement likely
9:00am - Highest testosterone secretion
10:00am - High alertness
2:30pm - Best coordination
3:30pm - Fastest reaction time
4:30pm - Greatest cardiovascular efficiency and
  muscle strength
6:30pm - Highest blood pressure
9:00pm - Melatonin secretion starts
10:30pm - Bowel movements suppressed.

Light, temperature, and other factors like jet lag and shift work will disconnect you from your internal clock. Your body has a set schedule for doing things at a certain time, give or take a couple hours. If your sleep times don't line up with the human circadian rhythm, it's harder to get good rest, no matter how tired you are.

Melatonin

Melatonin is our sleeping hormone. In order to make melatonin, I've read that you need to be asleep between three and six am. Most insomniacs are usually up during this time, and then we fall back asleep close to six am, which is when we need to wake up to get to work or deal with kids.

There are other factors that affect melatonin production. Exposure to sunlight also increases melatonin production, but most of us are stuck inside all day and night. Regular exercise in the mid to late afternoon also helps increase melatonin production, but many of us can only find time to exercise after kids are in bed and dishes are done, well after nine o'clock at night. We're often too tired to exercise at this time, and if we do, it makes it hard to fall asleep. Exercising in the mid or late afternoon helps to get rid of caffeine in our systems, and generally assists in the self-cleaning, but many working adults can't fit this in at this time.

The modern lifestyle also compromises our ability to make melatonin. For example, when we're out in the sun, we slather on the sunscreen or stay all covered up. When we come in, we jump of allowing the Vitamin D we've made to soak into our bodies.

The process of making melatonin starts at sundown, or when lights are dim. You need serotonin to make melatonin. Serotonin is a neurotransmitter that helps relax our brains. If you've used up all your serotonin dealing with your stressful day, then there's not enough left over to make sufficient melatonin. Without enough melatonin, the brain is overly active when it's time to fall asleep, and more wakefulness at night. Maybe you can't fall asleep for a long time. The result is less deep sleep and REM sleep. You wake up feeling like you haven't rested well.

One reason among many that caffeine is a problem for insomniacs is because it messes with internal clocks. Caffeine blocks adenosine receptors in the brain. Adenosine is the chemical we make that stops us from being wakeful at night. In effect, caffeine stimulates us because it slows down the normal action of the hormones that make us sleepy. That's why even though your caffeine buzz has worn off you still aren't sleepy at normal bedtime.

Stress Hormones - "Fight/Flight" in the Middle of the Night

Another problem for insomniacs is that we launch the flight/fight response when we're supposed to be sleeping. This is a chemical problem as well as a psychological one. At bed time, you start worrying if you'll be able to sleep, and how you'll function the next day. You start thinking about your husband who didn't wipe the counter down after he did the dishes, again. You have a co-worker who is badmouthing you behind your back. Your heart starts beating faster. All the hope you held for the night's sleep starts to dissipate. You may fall asleep anyway. But then you jerk awake suddenly and look at your watch, praying it's at least three o'clock, that you've slept at least three or four hours. Then you see that it's only midnight. You realize you've slept less than thirty minutes. You feel angry. Your heart is really racing now, and you feel kind of nauseous. You start getting warm, and soon you know getting back to sleep is impossible. That's cortisol, adrenaline (epinephrine) and noradrenaline (norepinephrine) facilitating physical reactions for sudden and significant muscular action. You might even get shaky and have tunnel vision. You feel hypersensitive to every noise and movement. Every snore, every creak, is amplified in your head.

You lie there, resisting getting up for as long as you can, hoping you'll at least rest. But then your feet get itchy and your legs get twitchy and the weight of the blankets drives you bonkers. That's your blood vessels dilating, liberating fat and glycogen for your muscles to use. Soon you can't resist the urge to dash out of the bed.

You go to the toilet, pace in the dark, trying not to turn on your computer or television. But you're really wide awake now, so one television show couldn't hurt. And online, there's a pair of shoes calling your name. You buy them and feel better for about five minutes. You keep surfing. You have a terrible headache but you're not sleepy. A couple hours pass. Your eyes are so tired that it's hard to focus to see the floor, but you're still not sleepy. You lie back in bed or on the sofa, but you still don't fall asleep. Your heart is still hammering. You imagine hearing the baby cry, a door slam, a gunshot, what have you. Every time you nod off you jerk back awake with nausea and a racing heart, with that feeling in the pit of your stomach like you've been falling off a cliff.

Our stress hormones are made by the adrenal glands, which are close to our kidneys. Cortisol is released when we're stressed and helps get sugar to our muscles quickly. Adrenaline, or epinephrine, gets you charged up for massive physical activity. It increases the flow of blood to your muscles, making your heart race, and also makes your lungs expand, so that you can breathe more deeply if needed. Noradrenaline, or norepinephrine, is a vasoconstrictor. It narrows your veins to help prevent bleeding to death in case you're injured. But this increases the workload on the heart to pump your blood through your body, and results in higher blood pressure and an increased heart rate.

Essentially, your anxiety about not falling asleep and any other problems on your mind have rocketed a big dose of stress hormones into your system right when you want to fall asleep. That's why your heart races and you get warm, agitated, nervous, angry. Just as you're supposed to be drifting into the land of Morpheus, your body activates the fight-flight response. If you could sprint away from a bear, you'd metabolize your stress hormones (use them up). But you don't do anything like that in the middle of the night, and your system is not working well enough to process the stress hormones quickly. So these chemicals course around your body for the rest of the night. You don't sleep deeply, or for long, and when you've slept just a couple hours, often you can't get back to sleep at all.

Why are you making these stress hormones when you're so tired? One reason is because you can't stop thinking about problems that you can't solve quickly. Hence you are constantly releasing stress hormones, all day long, so you literally stew in them. Another reason is because you're so tired. Your normal actions seem like very stressful activities to a body which no longer has time for self-repair and proper anti-stress hormone generation. Your body thinks you need the help to get the job done, and it shoots you full of the same stuff you'd use to pull a car off your child. The stress hormones help you be physically active—to engage in "flight" or "fight", but in the middle of the night in your safe bed, you certainly don't need them! You can't use them up because you're lying down. Maybe if you ran the treadmill for an hour, you'd burn them up, but then you'd never get back to sleep for sure. This is another example of how insomniacs are not aligned with our internal clocks.

In modern times, flight/fight responses have a wider range of behaviors. For example, angry, argumentative behavior, or social withdrawal and substance abuse. Although there is a short boost in your immune system after your flight/fight response is activated, a prolonged stress response is thought to result in chronic suppression of the immune system, which leaves you open to infections and other problems. Just another part of sleep deprivation's swath of destruction.

Insomniacs Don't Make Enough Helpful Chemicals
The third chemical complication insomniacs face is that we don't make enough helpful chemicals, and that's because we're busy making stress chemicals. Our adrenal glands also make DHEA, which is the

hormone from which we synthesize estrogen, progesterone and testosterone. As you probably know, these are the hormones that ensure the very survival of our species; we can't procreate without these.

In addition, testosterone happens to be the hormone that reduces stress in men. The adrenal gland also makes and releases oxytocin, which is the hormone that reduces stress in women. In other words, the release of these two hormones is what dissipates stress hormones. Both genders make both hormones and need them for various purposes, but for reducing stress, women need the oxytocin and men need testosterone. Men with too much oxytocin might get sluggish and women with too much testosterone might get even more stressed out. When we deprive ourselves of these happy hormones, women feel overwhelmed and men feel defeated. Dr. John Gray of Mars & Venus fame details this at length in his recent book <u>Venus on Fire, Mars on Ice: Hormonal Balance, the Key to Life, Love and Energy</u> (2010).

For women, oxytocin is released when we feel safe, nurtured and when we have the opportunity to nurture. For example, being appreciated for your hard work when your boss thanks you. Advising a friend on how to handle a problem, or receiving advice from a good friend, or getting a pedicure. Men need rest and successful problem solving opportunities to create testosterone. For example, knowing you did a good job when your boss thanks you. Watching the news on television for thirty minutes. Playing pool with your friends. Tinkering in the garage.

Mothers who work out of the home have a significant problem with high cortisol levels. Even if you're not employed at a boxing club, most working environments require women to release testosterone as part of what helps us get a job done quickly and efficiently. Nothing wrong with getting a job done well, but we may not be as relaxed as men when we do it. Then she goes home and has to start the busy night shift, so cortisol goes up even further. Cooking, dishes, chauffeuring, homework, whiny kids. By the time they're in bed, she's wiped out and flops in front of the tube. There's no other easy opportunity to decompress. The weekend comes; the dirty laundry is sky-high and her to-do list is intimidating.

Men, do you wonder why your women seem more stressed out than your mom was? It's because they are. Why are women more complicated now than in the past? Now that women work out of the home and for the most part, do the bulk of the work inside, their opportunities for oxytocin production are much more limited. I can't think of a single man my age who sacrifices as much personal time as the woman does for the sake of the household. More isolated from a community of women, we now look to our partners to take on that job of relieving our stress. Usually that doesn't work very well. Women are really good at keeping score in minute detail and resent having to sacrifice more than our husbands do.

Without enough testosterone, a man's stress levels rise quickly. He needs, as John Gray calls it, some "cave time" to replenish his testosterone stores. Men need thirty times more testosterone than women just to function normally. Women and men make the same amount of oxytocin, but a woman under stress depletes her supply more quickly. And of course, the last thing a stressed out woman does is find time to pamper herself, which is what she really needs to make more happy hormones.

Serotonin and dopamine are neurotransmitters that are really magical for us. They also help us make the hormone melatonin, which tells us it's time to shut down for the night. Serotonin is the neurotransmitter we use to relax and feel better when we're under stress. Women use more serotonin than men, since our brains are busier when we're stressed out. Women have more connective tissue between the left and right sides of our brains, and eight times the blood flow to our emotional center when we're even moderately stressed out (this is the limbic system: the hippocampus, which controls memory; the amygdala, which controls fear and love; and the hypothalamus, which is a gland that is thought to control the limbic system functions). Remember, without enough serotonin, we won't make enough melatonin. For men, without enough testosterone, they don't make dopamine, which gives them the motivation to problem solve their way through life's challenges.

Unfortunately just when you need it most, when you're sleep deprived, you stop making your happy chemicals in sufficient quantity. This is a particular issue for women, who have a harder time making serotonin than men do making dopamine. Not only is it harder to generate serotonin, but we make less of it for all the effort and we use it a lot faster. Hence women suffer more often from depression, anxiety and insomnia than men.

So why is it that we make less happy, helpful chemicals when we don't get enough sleep? When you learn how our chemistry works, you will have a much better understanding of how interconnected our minds and bodies are, how one problem cascades into a vicious cycle pretty quickly, and just how important it is to make healthy lifestyle choices for mind and body, and not rely on supplements and drugs, which don't adopt the necessary holistic approach to fixing your mind/body.

As I mentioned, the adrenal glands that make our stress hormones (cortisol, adrenaline, noradrenaline) also make our happy hormones. We are wired to prioritize survival over feeling good. This makes perfect sense: the body knows that feeling good won't matter if your head gets chopped off. The result is that we don't make as much DHEA (the hormone from which our procreation hormones come), or anti-stress hormones (testosterone and oxytocin) because the gland is busy making stress hormones for fight/flight.

Why Stress Hormones Stay Elevated

Most of us in western society aren't living through a war, so why are we stressed out? Modern lifestyle and eating habits cause so much of this trouble. We now keep ourselves in a condition when stress hormones are elevated chronically.

This is not what our bodies were intended for. We're designed for short bursts of elevated stress hormones. In the past we'd process the stress hormones fleeing or fighting the danger. The modern lifestyle presents us with situations that are continually out of our control--for example, traffic jams and noise and other annoyances of urban life, conflicts with co-workers and neighbors and spouses, no sense of life purpose and fulfillment, unhappy partners that we feel responsible to fix, children who have less respect for the knowledge and wisdom of their parents and elders and who pursue self-destructive habits very casually.

Modern privileges give us a sense of entitlement that lowers our tolerance for stressful situations. We don't have the cultural, spiritual, or ritual support to help us stop thinking about the problems we can't fix immediately. Hence our adrenal gland now works overtime. Plus, we don't use up the stress hormones with physical exertion like we used to, so they take longer to get out of our bodies. The result is that our bodies no longer have normal production of the happy chemicals.

Processed foods also interfere with the production of happy hormones by keeping stress hormones elevated. I'm not talking just about a microwave pizza: processed food is basically anything that has a label. It works like this: the processed food is either too sugary, or it doesn't have the natural fiber to slow down the release of sugar into the blood. We release insulin to store the sugar in our cells. (Over time we gain a bit of weight that seems ever harder to get rid of). When the insulin kicks in, our blood sugar goes down and down. One function of cortisol is to increase blood sugar (so we have quick energy for fight/flight). When our sugar goes back down we release cortisol. We get a strong urge to eat some bread or chocolate, and the cycle starts again.

You don't need to be diabetic to suffer from blood sugar fluctuations; some of the more noticeable symptoms are cravings for sugar and caffeine, and low energy or mood swings one to three hours after a meal. Why? Well, when our blood sugar is too low or too high, the brain chemistry is not appropriate for making serotonin or dopamine, so we feel even more agitated. We also don't make other feel-good neurotransmitters like endorphins and gamma-amino butyric acid (GABA). When blood sugar is low, a man can't make testosterone or dopamine, so these fluctuations can leave a man in a really crabby stupor. Without sufficient anti-stress chemicals to dissipate the elevated cortisol, your muscles stop burning fat for energy, and use sugar instead. Sugar is our emergency energy; fat gives us longer-lasting energy. With your muscles competing for sugar, there's just not enough sugar for your brain, so you crave more sugar.

If you eat within a few hours of bedtime, you start the cycle at bedtime, and have higher than natural release of cortisol in the middle of the night to alert you to low blood sugar. That's one reason a late or big meal keeps you up at night. Also, increased cortisol levels have been shown to cause a delay in the release of melatonin. Stabilizing blood sugar has been shown to get rid of many of the uncomfortable symptoms of menopause, in case you needed another incentive to get your diet in order!

It gets worse with age. For men, studies show an unprecedented drop in testosterone as they age. A forty-year old man today has the testosterone levels of a seventy-year old man thirty years ago! Experts believe this is caused by adrenal fatigue. Without enough testosterone to dissipate stress, a man ages much more quickly and can experience great dissatisfaction in life and numerous health problems. For women, an adrenal gland that's too busy making stress hormones won't be able to make enough estrogen once your ovaries slow down. Without the collaboration of estrogen and oxytocin, women feel increasing dissatisfaction and unhappiness. Once this happens, ain't no manicure-pedicure or spa day gonna fix you. With constantly elevated cortisol, the woman feels even more overwhelmed. Part of the stress response in women is activation of the emotional memory (lots of blood flow to the emotional center of the brain when stressed). So then we start cataloguing every bad thing that's happened to us, in specific, obsessive, detail, and it gets harder to shut off our brains at night and get into deep sleep.

If nothing I've said has sold you yet, then this will: sleep deprivation ages you and makes you fat. In laboratory rats, cortisol-induced collagen loss in the skin is ten times greater than in any other tissue![15] Premature aging, ladies, that no cream and surgery can fix. Eek! That's why your skin feels like it's sliding right off your face when you're exhausted. In fact, sleep deprivation has recently been shown to cause significant negative changes in our metabolism at a molecular level. The cells of someone slender and mostly healthy who doesn't get enough sleep look like the cells of someone who is overweight and sickly.[16]

To top it off, people who are sleep deprived are prone to storing fat, because the insulin sensitivity of your fat cells decreases significantly. Also, you don't make enough of something called leptin. This is the hormone that makes you feel full. This is accompanied by a rise in the levels of the hormone ghrelin, which tells you to keep eating. This would explain my insatiable urge to eat fatty foods during my time in the insomnia abyss. So if you're sleeping better, you will not only look better and feel better, but you might even lose some weight and be able to keep it off!

What's the big deal about deep sleep?

Deep sleep is the delta-wave sleep when our brains emit larger, slower waves. We are least responsive in deep sleep, so this is the sleep cycle when it's hardest to wake us up. Deep sleep makes up the smallest percentage of our total sleep in a seven or eight hour night.

How does the absence of deep sleep mess with our hormones?

---

[15] Houck, J.C. et al, "Induction of collagenolytic and proteolytic activities by anti-inflammatory drugs in the skin and fibroblast," Biochemical Pharmacology 17(10):2081-90 (October 1968).

[16] Based on a 2012 study by Eve Van Cauter, Professor of Medicine and Director of the Sleep Metabolism and Health Center at the University of Chicago. The study was published in the Annals of Internal Medicine, and cited by Luiza Ch. Savage, "The Sleep Crisis," Maclean's, (June 24, 2013), 49.

Enormously. Not only do we make critical growth hormone during deep sleep (for regeneration), but our body also breaks down proteins into the necessary amino acids to create happy brain chemicals.

These happy brain chemicals are fundamental to our normal functioning. Without them we feel really, really badly all the time. For example, tryptophan is extracted from proteins and moves into the brain to make serotonin. This relaxes the emotional part of the brain, and in turn a signal is sent to relax the adrenal glands so that we stop pumping out stress hormones. Dopamine gets made from the amino acid phenylalaline. Without dopamine we don't feel motivated to get up and face the day. GABA gets made from the amino acid glutamine, and this helps us enjoy our lives more; we can pour creativity and joy into even mundane tasks like washing dishes.

In a nutshell, these vital chemicals are made and do their important work of de-stressing us at night, when we are in the sleep phase called deep sleep. Without deep sleep, we get really messed up and miserable. We are not able to get off this wheel of fire unless we get deep sleep.

That's why the mere fact of existing felt like such an unbearable, purposeless burden during my long stretch of severe insomnia. No happy chemicals doing their important work at night.

My uncle used to tell me he wasn't sleeping at all in the hospital, and when I would check with the staff, they would tell me he was indeed sleeping or at least resting when they looked through his window. The problem was that he wasn't getting much or any of this magical deep sleep phase.

Let's say somebody listens to you complain about your life problems. Their reply? "Don't get so stressed out about small things. Don't take everything so personally. Don't be so negative. Why are you still worrying about this? Just shake it off!" Well, when you are no longer making enough happy brain chemicals, you are no longer able to shake anything off. Obsession, anxiety and paranoia work their tentacles into your thoughts. You may long to be less anxious, but you find that you simply are not able to. Why? You need your happy brain chemicals to do this, and you no longer make them in sufficient quantity to function normally in life. Without your happy chemicals, you can't face the problems life presents to every single person.

What is Gratitude, Chemically?

Your grandmother taught you that counting your blessings made you feel better. In contemporary holistic healing circles, you call it "raising your vibration." It is said that gratitude is the emotion that lifts your "vibration" to the highest it can get in the physical world. There's also a chemical, physiological way to put it: gratitude helps you relax and fall back asleep because it generates a surge of happy chemicals that does indeed dissipate stress hormones. That warm fuzzy feeling or surge you get when you think of someone you really love, something you enjoy or are proud of or are excited about, is not just psychological and spiritual. That is your body chemistry at work. When we have enough happy and helpful chemicals in our bodies, we can make miracles happen, like fixing our insomnia. It is the best, easiest and fastest way to make miracles happen. The sophistication, precision, and complexity of our internal chemistry can never be duplicated by pharmaceuticals. Our bodies are really, really amazing.

Insomnia's Link to Hormone Deficiency

I know now that many of my insomnia-induced problems were also symptoms of hormone deficiency: accelerated aging, depression and anxiety, panic attacks, indigestion, increase in blood pressure, difficulty breathing, heart palpitations, joint pain and muscle aches, inflammation, increased sensitivity to pain, vertigo & dizzy spells, food and environmental sensitivities and more. My thyroid problems may also have been attributable to high cortisol levels, for the thyroid regulates your metabolism during non-stressful times, and begins to under-function when it never has the opportunity to do its job.

But once I was sleeping again, these problems went away within a few months!

Elevated cortisol and lower levels of helpful happy chemicals made me crave, incessantly, heavy and crappy food. I gained a pile of weight quickly, thanks to the cycle of sugar addiction. Ice cream, processed meat, and copious quantities of chocolate were my vices, and these are filled with toxic chemicals that certainly placed a burden on my liver. A more toxic body turns into a breeding ground for Candida, which migrates from your intestines all over the body. Excess Candida is associated with chronic infections, sore throat, stuffed nose, and frequent illness.

I also experienced cycles of profound exhaustion and depression during a single day. Most insomniacs will agree that mornings are the worst time. You are certain you cannot go on; you will not have the capacity to simply exist for the next few hours. You don't have any will to live. Some of this may be attributed to sleep inertia, a condition when you are groggy and clumsy after an abrupt awakening. Scientists think sleep inertia happens when you're awakened from deep sleep (slow-wave NREM-3), or awakened when your body temperature is still low. But for insomniacs it's a lot worse than having slow reflexes and a thick tongue. Non-insomniacs might have a strong urge to go back to sleep. The insomniac can't shut down her brain anyway and just wants to collapse, curl up and die.

Then I'd perk up in the late morning, feel peppy and happy, crash in the pit of despair again in the middle of the afternoon, with the cycle repeated one more time before my kids' bedtime at about eight o'clock. Another physical symptom was the racing heart. My resting heart rate was often over ninety beats per minute. During the crashes I mentioned above, sometimes it would skyrocket to 120 and I'd be very faint. I'd also experience what I later understood to be panic attacks—difficulty breathing, fainting spells, inability to make simple decisions.

Yet when I practiced a Russian method of breath holding (Buteyko Breathing Method), where I slowed my inhalation to once per minute, I was able to slow my heart rate back down within a few minutes and stop a panic attack in progress. I didn't need any pills, therapy or any psychoanalysis: the problem had simple chemical origins (the symptoms of panic attack are caused by a sudden release of adrenaline) and a simple physical solution. The technique is something like inhale for ten seconds, hold for twenty seconds, exhale for thirty seconds. This method posits that shallow and too frequent inhalation (hyperventilation) hampers all bodily functions. Once you are able to hold your breath for more than two minutes, you experience significant health improvements in all areas of your physiology, including a reduction in the number of hours of sleep needed to function optimally.

This was one of the results my husband reported. During this time he trained to hold his breath for about two minutes, and not only did he improve his vision so that he no longer needed reading glasses, but he started getting up, feeling well rested, at 5:30am, on less than seven hours sleep, which for him is really unusual. Having been an active soldier, he has had turbulent "battle" dreams for as long as I have known him, yet while he was training with this breathing method, he stated that his sleep seemed very deep and undisturbed by dreams. These results require ongoing training however, about an hour a day. When he stopped practicing, his vision worsened again and he went back to his ten hours a night of sleep.[17]

The fact that you can train yourself to relax, and that your intention and habit have a major impact on your health is shown is studies that measure the blood pressure of adults who observe the afternoon siesta. When people knew they were going to take a nap, they experienced a large reduction in blood pressure when zoning out for their afternoon nap. When the people hadn't *planned on* having a nap, they didn't experience that big drop in blood pressure during the daytime onset of sleep.[18] That's how strong the mind-body connection is. This is not new-age fluff. Our hormones are the link. The siesta habit has been associated with a significant reduction in coronary mortality, and this siesta-induced reduction in cardiovascular stress is thought to play a role.[19] How wonderful, that an afternoon nap can do so much to keep our hearts strong and healthy! Inexpensive and fun.

Your Job is to Fix Your Chemical Problem

If I can do it, and the afternoon nappers worldwide can do it, then you can too. One of your principal jobs is to realign with your internal clock so you can restore a normal hormone supply/release. This is how you teach yourself to sleep again. You help your body to make the right chemicals at the right time. You help it make more of the good stuff. You keep your body clean to help it experience and process life with the least amount of effort. This is not instantaneous; it takes practice and time. Be patient during your metamorphosis, instead of getting anxious and popping a sleeping pill or anti-anxiety

---

[17] Hard as it is to believe in scalpel-happy and pill-happy North America, but the Buteyko Breathing Method is well respected in Russia, Ukraine and other CIS countries as a cure for many ails, particularly asthma and other lung conditions. You can find many videos on YouTube as well as free information and books online.

[18] Zaregarizi, Mohammad Reza, "Effects of Exercise & Daytime Sleep on Human Haemodynamics: With Focus on Changes in Cardiovascular Function during Daytime Sleep Onset," (LAP LAMBERT Academic Publishing, 2012).

[19] Naska, A., et al, "Siesta in healthy adults and coronary mortality in the general population," Archives of Internal Medicine 167(2):296-201 (2007).

pill during the night.

Now that you know sleeping aids prevent you from reaching deep sleep, I hope you will hesitate before taking any more pills! Remember, the more you sleep, the more you can sleep.

The practice of Banish / Gratitude trained me to fall back asleep again or calm down after waking up suddenly. I didn't fall asleep quickly; sometimes it took a couple hours, but even that was progress after not being able to fall back asleep at all. My pattern went something like this: sleep thirty minutes, up an hour, sleep an hour, up a couple hours, etc. After a couple months of steadily improving sequential hours of sleep, I was able to sleep two or three hours in a row each night, and deeply. In about nine months I was able to sleep two or sometimes even three hours in a row *twice* per night. Sleep two or three hours, up for an hour, sleep another two hours, awake thirty minutes, doze restlessly for an hour. During the next year I slept a few hours, was up for an hour, then I'd sleep three or four hours straight. Today, which is three years after my worst condition, I sleep five or six hours straight, sometimes seven. I wake up with energy and don't have any difficulty getting out of bed or starting my day. I don't need a shower or a coffee to wake myself up. I don't need a nap in the afternoon.

This might not sound like a heck of a lot of sleep, but remember, I was sleeping less than five hours *a week* when I hit rock bottom, let alone five hours per night!

So what can you do to get your internal chemistry lined up behind your efforts to restore healthy sleep? In the next chapter, I will share what worked for me.

Summary

- Our society undervalues sleep because the way it helps us is not widely understood.

- Sleeping aids aren't chemically able to make us sleep better. They even prevent us from going into deep-sleep. Sleeping aids have bad side effects and cause new health problems for the insomniac.

- Insomniacs make stress hormones when we should be sleeping and we don't make enough happy chemicals because we maintain high stress hormone levels.

- This chemical problem means the less you sleep, the more you lose the ability to sleep. The more you sleep, the more you restore your ability to sleep.

- You can fix your insomnia by teaching yourself to make more happy chemicals and to release fewer stress hormones.

5 BE YOUR OWN CHEMIST

For the insomniac, the laboratory of your body means that the less you sleep, the less you are *able* to sleep. The more you sleep, the more you are *able* to sleep. You need to sleep to start sleeping better. But how can you get more sleep? You can't fall asleep. You can't stay asleep. The longer you've been sleep deprived, the harder it is. So how do you teach yourself to sleep again?

The answers are not pharmaceutical, that's for sure. Sleeping is a habit you train yourself to accomplish. You start by being your own chemist. Indeed, as I described in the previous chapter, you are a *remarkable* chemist. Your body is your one-stop laboratory, and changing your chemistry by yourself is faster and more effective than a pill prescribed by a doctor.

Your ingredients are your thoughts, your actions, your food. Your experiments are risk free without a single negative side effect. The rules are simple and easy to remember: garbage in, garbage out. Good stuff in, good stuff out.

How do you adjust your body's chemistry? You make psychological and physical adjustments to your life so that you

- Don't make stress hormones when you should be sleepy or sleeping,
- Make more helping & happy chemicals,
- Keep your body clean to conserve your energy for your body's self-healing work, and
- Stay patient so you can give your body the necessary time to accomplish this goal.

#1: Be Mindful of Your Thoughts

Number one: start a disciplined mental practice where you count your blessings instead of your gripes. How do you do this? We talked about this earlier.

1. Focus on what's good instead of what's bad about your life.
2. Stop judging yourself, your family and friends, and everyone else.

Sounds hard, huh? In fact we practice such selective intention all the time elsewhere in our lives. When you're at a buffet, you choose the food you like, not the food that makes you sick. You don't pick a slum for a vacation destination; you pick a nice place where you think you'll have some adventure, rest and fun. After going to the bathroom, would you leave your bottom dirty instead of wiping it off and washing up? Of course not; it's unthinkable. Treat your mind and spirit with the same automatic respect, courtesy and care by choosing to keep your thoughts clean and healthy. During the night, choose the thoughts that let you fall asleep, and fall back asleep when you wake up.

The Only Thing You Control is Your Thoughts

The practice of non-judgment is also called forgiveness in some circles. When you stop judging yourself and others about everything, you are forgiving everyone, of everything, all the time. Not because you condone their actions, but because you don't *control* their actions. The only thing you control is your thoughts. This is what it means to be compassionate and turn the other cheek. You don't have to be a doormat, or tolerate abusive behavior, but you're no longer in a position where you can afford to let the actions of others disturb your sleep. Being more loving and compassionate to those you love and also to strangers has a huge chemical impact: your happy hormones get generated because you feel more in control. That's because instead of a knee-jerk reaction, you are pausing to choose your emotional response to situations. You also feel happier because you are giving something very important--love, compassion, kindness, understanding--to those around you.

We don't know what despair or illusion leads to the actions and words of others. Maybe they regret being mean to you, and they feel badly about it. Maybe everyone you interact with feels as terrible as you, so be grateful that things aren't worse. If everyone around me felt as nasty and hateful and paranoid as I felt in my darkest moments, we'd already have self-destructed as a species.

The fact that my family blew off my condition so easily and thoroughly was devastating to my self-esteem. It made me feel worthless. When I opened up to them, infrequently as it was, they really didn't want to hear it, and they didn't want to be involved in the solution. It was only after my uncle's death that they began to treat insomnia as a health crisis. They simply didn't know better; they didn't mean to hurt me.

This type of unconditional forgiveness isn't a natural part of our overachiever, greedy culture, where we think that others are always trying to take things from us, and that there's not enough happiness to go around. This basic Christian teaching goes completely unpracticed moment-by-moment. Yet that's where it's needed most, is in the moment. Each thought, each interaction. Stop complaining and criticizing for your own sake, so that *you* feel better. It's not about anyone else, only you. It's the ultimate self-help act: when you let go of judgment, and when you stop trying to control others' thoughts and actions, you feel immense relief.

Why? Why would this make you feel better? The answer is simple and chemical: you're not making stress hormones from worrying about something. When you're not worrying, you give your body the time it needs to make the other chemicals that help you feel better and that fix your body. Even better, when you choose to focus on the positive, when you are grateful or happy or proud of someone or something, you stimulate the release of your happy hormones that dissipate stress hormones.

Why is this discipline so powerful that it makes it to the top of my list, way ahead of lavender oil and no television in the bedroom? Because it helps you naturally sedate those emotions like anger and fear that engage your flight/fight response in the middle of the night.

Science has long since proven what we know instinctively: that our bodies and minds are inseparably linked. Science has a name for the link: it's called hormones. It's called body chemistry. When we change the mind we change the body. When we change the body we change the mind. In fact, the fastest way to change the body is to change the mind! It can take hours to wind down after your heart starts racing. Frequently I was never able to wind down at all. The trick is prevent your heart from starting to race in the first place, and the only answer is to control your thoughts.

There are a number of other benefits of this practice that

contribute to restored sleep health, too. For example, during prayer / meditation / guided meditation, your active or "beta" brain waves become relaxed "alpha" waves. So this is a way to rest your brain even if you can't sleep. Do not underestimate how important and helpful this kind of rest is; I frequently was able to relax deeply even if I could not sleep, and sometimes it was the only break I had from the torment of my exhaustion and anxiety. Another huge plus is that people who meditate generally need less sleep.[20] In other words, your sleep becomes more efficient. If you're tired of spending eight hours in bed, but you're not sleeping well and you still feel exhausted, this practice may be just what you need. You'll be able to spend less time in bed.

If you can teach yourself to be more peaceful, you will feel better, you will sleep more deeply, and you will also need less sleep. It's a win-win all around without a single bad side effect. Package that in a bottle and sell it!

Colin Tipping is a writer and speaker that has outlined a simple four-step process to help us be mindful of our thoughts. If you can pull this out when you're tempted to stew in self-criticism or judgment, you will have immediate change in your thinking:

1. I look at what I have created.
2. I notice my judgments and feelings but love myself anyway.
3. I am willing to see the perfection in this situation.
4. I choose peace.[21]

If this kind of analysis is too much for you at night, which it often was for men when I felt really terrible, you can try something a lot easier. Thich Nhat Hanh, in his book Peace is Every Step, outlines a number of easy and active meditations. Instead of emptying your mind or working through your problems, you think about breathing. Below, I quote just one of many simple and effective breathing exercises he provides in this short and easy-to-read book. With each inhalation and exhalation, you repeat a mantra:

---

[20] Kaul, Prashant et al, "Meditation acutely improves psychomotor vigilance and may decrease sleep need," Behavioral and Brain Functions 6:47 (2010).
[21] Colin Tipping, Radical Forgiveness: A Revolutionary Five-Stage Process to Heal Relationships, Let Go of Anger and Blame, and Find Peace in Any Situation (Sounds True, 2009)

Breathing in, I calm my body. *[inhale]*
Breathing out, I smile. *[exhale]*
Dwelling in the present moment *[inhale]*
I know this is a wonderful moment. *[exhale]*[22]

Humor Helps Us Change the Mental Channel

One way to improve your attitude is with humor. Laughter helps you change your mental channel, and can pull you out of complain-and-whine mode really quickly and easily, without any effort or analysis. There is of course a chemical explanation! Gelatologists (yes, there is a name for those who study laughter; go ahead and laugh if you like) tell us that laughter signals acceptance in a group. Laughter is how we demonstrate positive interactions with others. Laughter is how we express excitement, inward joy, and happiness.

Chemically this manifests in reduced cortisol and adrenaline levels, the release of endorphins that can relieve some physical pain, a boost in antibody-producing cells, and an enhancement of the effectiveness of T-cells, leading to a stronger immune system.

As we know, children laugh a lot more than adults; I read on Wikipedia that babies laugh about three hundred times per day, and adults only around twenty times per day! Burdened with the complexities of adult life, we envy them this freedom and pleasure. When I snap at my kids, I often feel just terrible afterwards. As a Course in Miracles student, I am devoted to practicing non-judgment and love in my day-to-day interactions with not only family, friends and colleagues, but also strangers. This active meditation is the most important part of my day, every day. When I mess up and give into a tantrum or pettiness, I am very self-critical. I, of all people, should have known better, and should be able to put my walk where my talk is. And yet no matter how crabby I've been, my children always accept my apology instantly, and always have a smile and hug ready for me. They just bounce back in a way that inspires and amazes me. It's a miracle to watch them in action, and it teaches me that by taking myself just a little less seriously I feel a lot better. If they can forgive me so easily, then I can forgive myself, too.

Many television dramas today are extremely dark and violent, filled with frustrated, ultra-serious humans unable to solve their problems and unable to relate peacefully to anyone in any of their circles. I'm a sucker for a good storytelling, and the quality of television writing

---

[22] Thich Nhat Hanh, Peace is Every Step, 10.

today is superior to what you find in feature films. Hence I am easily hooked on television dramas, especially cop, lawyer, sci-fi, futuristic, and fantasy shows. Today, that's dozens of shows, and for this reason I don't subscribe to cable television service or I'd never get anything done. I stream a few shows occasionally, but when I feel myself getting more tired or not sleeping as well as I like to, I go on a diet and stop watching stressed-out people cope with stress.

Instead, I'll have a look at something lighter or happier. I recommend picking out a favorite funny show that you enjoyed when you were younger. I Love Lucy, Gilligan's Island, The Three Stooges. Looney Tunes. Or something else that makes you laugh. I love 30 Rock. That show has made me laugh harder than I ever thought I could. Give yourself permission to take twenty minutes to laugh during a comedy show, and you will reward yourself instantaneously with all sorts of happy chemicals. Even better: get out and see a live comedy show. A recent comedy project that I have found to be hilarious and helpful is the Spiritual Comedy Festival. Many of the videos are available for free on the internet at http://www.spiritualcomedyfestival.com.

#2: Take Appropriate Action to Solve or Come to Terms With Your Problems

Your first step, in your chemical experiment, is training your mind to count your blessings instead of your gripes. This makes lots of happy chemicals and helps keep the stress hormones at bay. Secondly, if you have some issues that keep your mind in turmoil, you need to take action to bring about resolution so that you can be more peaceful.

Positive thinking can help you feel a lot better but it doesn't solve your problems. That's what action is for. That's what daytime is for. If you don't take action, then you leave yourself open to night-time worry. Worry serves no purpose; it is merely stretching out fear over time. It's a total waste of your potential. Chemically, worry results in fewer chemicals for regeneration and restoration.

In the middle of the night, when you should be resting your tired brain, your worst fears rise most quickly to the surface. Issues and projections that you can keep at bay during the day come out storming. This also has chemical underpinnings: if you haven't reached deep sleep or REM sleep, your brain can't do any self-repair, cleaning and organizing. That's why you kind of feel crazy in the middle of the night when you're not sleeping, night after night.

Why do people complain so much? Especially women, my gawd. It's not because we like to complain, even though this may be true since some of us are chemically addicted to our own drama. It's because we want stress relief. Being steeped in stress hormones makes us feel terrible. We want someone or something to help us handle the problems that are beyond our control and causing our fight/flight response to stay launched. But the stress isn't going anywhere; you must change your thoughts and actions. When you take action to help yourself, you are reasserting your control over a problem, and you are helping yourself make and release helpful chemicals.

If you're hiding big lies, if you've got serious financial problems, personal problems, career problems, chronic pain and sickness, a delinquent or sick child, grief and other serious trauma, or any of the other big life change issues, it is time to take some action to initiate the healing, resolution or change that you desire.

That action may be deciding to surrender your attempts to control a situation that you do not control, like a struggling adult child. At minimum you need some work/life balance: you must find some personal time to decompress your brain or your stress and anxiety will carry through to bedtime. This balance should not be optional. Work/life balance is a much better investment in your health than expensive health care premiums and prescription drugs.

No one's life is easy and problem free. It is normal to have ups and downs in all areas of our life—personal, professional, social. This is not going to change. If you're a sociopath, then maybe big life problems don't bother you, but most people get stressed out consciously and subconsciously, and thus we let the big life problems keep us up at night. If you take appropriate action during the day they will interfere less with your sleep. You are responsible for initiating a solution so that you can support your primary goal of restoring healthy sleep. Maybe you can't fix the problem, or maybe it's going to take quite a bit of time, like dealing with grief.

Regardless, once you take some action, you will feel immense relief. Why? Because self-nurturing makes women release oxytocin, and facing a problem squarely makes men release testosterone. That's what makes us feel better, our happy hormones.

This doesn't mean you need to aim for a lottery win so you can quit an unsatisfying job. Make your action reasonable; make your goals small and achievable, so you can frequently pat yourself on the back for accomplishing them.

- Book an appointment for counseling.
- Call a help line.
- Go to the library to take out some self help books and CDs, or watch some gurus or speakers you like on YouTube.
- Join a grief or addiction support group.
- Come clean about your truth.
- Exercise four times per week.
- Pray.
- Acknowledge that you need something, like work-life balance.
- Ask for the help you need.
- Admit you made a mistake and ask for forgiveness.
- Accept that your house will not stay clean for more than ten minutes after you've cleaned it until your children are older.
- Declare an intention to be unbotherable by the judgments of others.
- Declare that you will stop comparing yourself to others.
- Set a family meeting or schedule an appointment with your boss or a colleague so you can state what is bothering you.
- Telephone a family member to explain why something he or she said or did made you feel deeply hurt.
- Write down a list of goals, actions and a timeline.
- Keep track of your progress and surround yourself with supportive listening materials.
- Create a vision board.
- Research your next career path for ten minutes each day.
- Find a community of like-minded people so you have someone to talk to.
- Meet with your spiritual guide or counselor.
- Be reasonable about your to-do list! Cut yourself some slack.

Some action, even if just baby steps, can help give you immense relief at night. It will be that much easier to choose thoughts that help you sleep when you know that you've done something during the day to solve your problems. If you would rather worry and stew at night than take any action, this means you are not prioritizing your health. You are choosing to stay awake and suffer in misery rather trying to help yourself. Your suffering can only make you sicker, and has no ability to make you sleep or get stronger.

If you feel that you deserve to suffer, this is a sign of depression; it is time to seek help right away. You do not deserve to suffer! Your emotions are your guide, and when you feel badly, this is your body's way of telling you it's time to make some changes. Often it's hard to see through your own muddle; seek external help.

Help Yourself Make Happy Hormones

Even if you can't fix your problems, you can still engage in activities that stimulate the release of our happy hormones, oxytocin and testosterone. For men, this needs to include time to rest, private time, and opportunities for successful problem solving. Ladies, don't complain when your man wants to go to the gym twice a week even though you rarely get out, or if he would rather mow the lawn rather than snuggle with you. He is all the better for it, and with more testosterone he is better equipped to help you make oxytocin.

For women, this means time to give and receive nurturing. Gents, don't roll your eyes at your wife for going over the same problems over and over with her friends, or begrudge her that new pair of shoes. She needs opportunities to feel listened to and pampered. Plus--ye gods--if she can't talk to her friends she'll expect you to be the one who listens and empathizes.

People should encourage their partners to invest their time and energy in some activities that help them produce and release happy hormones. It's not enough to expect the annual two-week vacation to sort you out; take these small actions to make sure you keep a regular supply of happy hormones in your body, because you need to use them all the time. What else can you do? Lots. Go to the gym; set a new goal for exercise; take some down time to snuggle; set some time aside for girly talk or bro-mance.

For both men and women, some kind of volunteer service is a superb way to stimulate your happy hormones. Women get the immense satisfaction of knowing they are helping people who really need it. Men get the immense satisfaction of knowing they are doing something noble and important to save their community. But you also get to walk away after your shift and not be chronically bogged down in problems you can't fix permanently and politics that are stressful. Also, unlike with your family, friends and colleagues, you won't be tempted to complain and get agitated about what you're not getting in return for your hard work. You've heard the phrase "it's in giving that we receive?" There's a chemical reason for it. When we provide volunteer service, we're usually happy to give for the sake of giving alone, and chemically, that's exactly why it feels so good.

The modifications I have suggested so far are extremely significant in preventing yourself from launching the flight-fight response in the middle of the night, and for generating more of your own happy chemicals. Remember, the more happy chemicals you make, the more melatonin you make and the easier it is to fall and stay asleep according to the rhythm of your internal clock. It makes it that much easier to build up the habit of sleeping again.

#3: Keep Your Body Healthy with Diet and Exercise

The insomniac also needs to be conscious of diet and exercise and follow some guidelines that help you keep your body healthy. When your body is healthy, you are much more efficient and productive chemically. These physical changes are easier to implement because they don't require that you do anything as hard as give up a grudge you hold dear. The rewards manifest immediately and are very motivating. Even better, because our minds and bodies are one big chemical system, the physical changes support the psychological changes.

Get Off Drugs

Firstly, get off drugs. I hope you are already planning to wean yourself off of sleeping aids, because they will hinder all attempts to sleep deeply. They don't allow you to align with your internal clock, and to boot they depress your body functions, such as preventing you from making helpful chemicals. If possible, you should also consider weaning yourself off of anti-anxiety medication if you can, because for many, the real commitment to mental / spiritual discipline will fill this gap. These heavy drugs don't allow you to align with your body's own gentle natural rhythms and chemistry. Frankly, some of the research I've done about how pharmaceuticals engage your chemistry suggests that many of the pills we commonly take for reducing blood pressure, cholesterol, and for pain management reduce your body's production of the basic sex hormones as well as your anti-stress hormones!

Then there's the illegal heavy drugs; I don't have any experience with these but I have heard that these can cause both insomnia and hypersomnia, where the user sleeps too much. I know people who use illegal drugs, and in my observation these interfere greatly with your internal clock, and exaggerate the extreme traits of your personality.

From my personal experience, marijuana is not a hypnotic (sleep inducer) at all. In fact, much the opposite for me. Once I ate a "space brownie" to gauge whether THC would help with insomnia. Unfortunately I spent the next terrible fifty hours vibrating in vigilant paranoia! I will never use marijuana again; it was very counterproductive for me. I've heard that weed can have this effect on high-strung people, but my husband is laid back and he also became very paranoid under the influence of marijuana.

I have also heard that most street marijuana is grown with fertilizers that contain speed and crack, and that paranoia after using marijuana is much more common than it was twenty or thirty years ago. However, Massimo Mazzucco, an Italian filmmaker, has an excellent documentary about the potential benefits of organic, natural marijuana.

There are plenty of strong legal drugs that the insomniac should cut out of his or her diet; the first of these is good ole caffeine. In addition to the chemical problems I mentioned earlier, whereby caffeine interferes with the chemicals that prevent wakefulness, caffeine is also is linked to raised cortisol levels.

I have some additional concerns about caffeine. When you're an insomniac, you already have unmanageable ups and downs during the day. Caffeine, which kicks you into overdrive and is followed by a crash, makes the amplitude of these swings much greater. It's that much more exhausting; it makes getting through the day that much more physical work. The jitters and crash require physical bandwidth that you don't have anymore. Also, sleeplessness is much easier to handle without caffeine. If you're up at night, you're more relaxed and mellow without caffeine. It is much easier to ride the emotionally difficult times in the middle of the night. When you're caffeinated, even if you're no longer buzzed, the crazy emotions of the pre-dawn hours are exaggerated.

Giving up your favorite Starbucks delicacy might seem too masochistic, but remember, it only takes seventeen days to form a new habit. If you are truly committed to improving your sleep, your efforts will be quickly rewarded with more patience, more energy and better rest. It only takes a few days to get used to life without caffeine.

Plan to go cold turkey on a weekend so you can manage the headaches more easily. Usually caffeine withdrawal headaches only last for one or two days. Drink a lot of water, take a cold shower, and get out in the fresh air for a walk to help with headaches. Have a cup of green or black tea to tide you over, but plan to cut those out too.

Diet pills and decongestants stimulate your brain and cause insomnia, so avoid them! Some diet pills contain powerful stimulants like caffeine and/or epinephrine (the latter makes your heart beat faster so you burn more calories). Decongestants contain pseudoephedrine or phenylephrine. Both of these are vasoconstrictors, which means they shrink your blood vessels and thus increase your blood pressure and heart rate. If I'm really suffering from a cold and take a decongestant, I do not even fall asleep; that's how powerful they are.

Alcohol might make you drowsy at first, but when it metabolizes you get some rebound sleeplessness. That's why you might go to bed tipsy but sleep very fitfully, or wake up at 3am and not fall asleep afterward. If you're drinking too much or even an extra glass of wine at night to help calm down, this is not going to help you sleep. Alcohol reduces the quality of your sleep. Have your glass of vino earlier on with food, but don't have more than a couple glasses. I don't think it's a good idea to drink more than a couple times per week.

Smoking also makes you sleep lighter and have reduced REM sleep. In fact, smokers can experience increased wakefulness due to nicotine withdrawal in the middle of the night. Save your wine and smokes for when you're sleeping better; your body is just too sensitive for the extra load when you're an insomniac. Your self-cleaning systems aren't working optimally when you're chronically sleep deprived, so your ability to clean out toxins like alcohol and cigarette chemicals is compromised.

Cut Out Processed Foods / Sugary Foods

Eating healthy unprocessed foods in light meals is a really big deal for someone with sleeping problems. Remember the rules of the chemical game? Garbage in, garbage out. Good stuff in, good stuff out. It's not about making you thinner, preventing cancer, getting rid of health problems, or even feeling better--all of which are awesome side effects of eating less processed and sugary food. For a person with sleeping problems, when you eat unprocessed foods you create the right chemical environment for sleeping. With stabilized blood sugar, you prevent chronic stress hormone secretion and you free up your body to make more happy chemicals. Processed food either has too much sugar, or releases the sugar into your bloodstream too quickly. You crank out insulin to sort yourself out, which makes your blood sugar go down quickly. This launches a secretion of cortisol, which starts the cycle all over. The net result is that your adrenal gland stays busy making stress hormones and thus makes fewer happy hormones, and you get both fatter and sicker.

What exactly is processed food? I recently heard an interview with well-known endocrinologist and obesity doctor, Robert Lustig, on Science Friday where he sums it up neatly: "If it has a label, it's garbage. Total garbage."[23] Processed flour, sugary food, prepackaged foods, canned foods, restaurant food and basically any grocery item with a label is loaded with sugars and chemicals that slow down digestion, affect our immune system and affect our hormone production. Not only are the added sugars a problem: once a food is removed from its natural fiber environment, the sugar gets delivered to your bloodstream too quickly. Think real apple vs. fruit rollup.

Start taking the time to prepare your own food. This is an investment of time, not a waste of time. You don't ever need to feel hungry eating lighter; in fact, you will be surprised at how full you are. One principal advantage is the ease of digestion: you won't ever drop into the post-meal food coma. Gas and constipation are much reduced.

Can you eat sweet stuff? Sure. As long as it comes in an unprocessed form, and if you need the chocolate mousse with whipped cream, save it for once a week. Load up on ripe fresh fruit. The more colors the better. If you put a big bowl of fresh fruit salad and a chocolate cake in front a group of small children, they will always choose the fruit. It's colorful, juicy, and comes in little awesome shapes that are easy for little fingers to practice pincer action on. It's fun to eat. They completely ignore the cake--it looks boring, chalky, and is the color of poop.

My kids like to wear their raspberries, one on each finger and thumb, and eat them methodically and joyfully; it's the cutest thing

---

[23] Dr. Lustig was interviewed on NPR's Science Friday weekly radio program on January 11, 2013. He is the author of Fat Chance: Beating the Odds Against Sugar, Processed Food, Obesity, and Disease, (Hudson Street Press, 2012).

ever. Unfortunately we train this wonderful instinct for fresh, juicy fruits out of children, and by the time your kids are about seven, most will go for the cake first. If like me, you need your chocolate fix, then at least eat a smaller piece of organic chocolate instead of a big cheap chocolate bar.

Notice how diabetics don't have problems eating fruit? That's because the sugar in the fruit doesn't make your insulin levels spike. But, cook the fruit, dry the fruit, or process it into fruit roll-ups, and you have a higher "glycemic load." Unprocessed food has a lower "glycemic load," meaning how quickly sugar from the food gets to the bloodstream. Most fruits have a low glycemic load (except bananas) because they are mostly water. That's why dried fruit gets to your bloodstream faster.

Type two diabetes is one of the fastest diseases to cure with diet changes for the reasons I cite above. Even something as simple as cooking your oatmeal from the whole oat groat versus the quick-serve rolled oats makes a significant difference on glycemic load. It's twenty minutes versus two minutes, but it makes an enormous difference in your wellbeing and that of your children. You will be thinner and feel better.

The most important action is to cut out unprocessed food, like fast food and frozen pizzas and dinners. Basically, uncooked fruit and vegetables should make up more than half what goes into your mouth. Without sweet and oily sauces. Make your own salad dressing quickly with olive oil, lemon or vinegar, and salt / spices. Base more of your meals on potatoes and yams and fewer on pasta and rice.

But if you can, also keep your diet clean and natural. Buy organic where possible, at least for the "dirty dozen", which are the most contaminated with pesticide.

- Peaches
- Apples
- Sweet Bell Peppers
- Celery
- Nectarines
- Strawberries
- Cherries
- Pears
- Grapes

- Spinach
- Lettuce
- Potatoes

If possible, stick to organic dairy and meat. Genetically modified food and pesticide-fed animals create gut bacteria that interferes with digestion. A less expensive solution is to reduce or eliminate animal flesh and animal products while you're learning to sleep again.

Some people may think they don't have enough money to eat unprocessed or organic food, but in fact, when you are eating better food, and unprocessed food, you actually end up eating less. That's because the food, having more nutrients, is more satiating. Also, your body won't go through the sugars of unprocessed foods as fast, so you crave less and don't get hungry again as quickly. You will also be more careful about not wasting what's in your fridge.

I heard a recent study about the level of minerals in organic and non-organic food being similar. This study was misleading and probably funded by someone who stood to gain from the publicity. When you take a look at some of the chemistry involved you will see why: Monsanto's popular Round Up herbicide is a metal chelator, meaning that it binds metals. How does this interact with plants? Well, dirt has some free-form metals (these we call minerals). These are molecules that have a positive or negative charge. The herbicide makes the free-form metal stick to the herbicide molecule.

The result? The mineral is then unavailable for the plants to absorb, so the weeds starve to death. But the crops are genetically modified to survive mineral deprivation, so they don't die. They may not be very healthy, but they survive the herbicide. The herbicide also starves the ground's bacteria of minerals, so these critters also die and don't give their good poop to the plant and dirt. The soil becomes able to sustain only the plant that's genetically modified to withstand mineral deprivation. When you hear stories about produce grown fifty years ago having six times the nutrients that the same produce has today, this is why.

Sometimes when people start a vegan or raw-food diet, they eat too many nuts and too much oil. Avoid overloading on these; they are slower to digest and can undo some of the benefits you are aiming for.[ii] If you want something heavier, eat a bit of coconut oil, some avocado, or eat soaked nuts, but not more than four tablespoons a day. What's a soaked nut? Stick the nuts in a jar of water for eight hours (or overnight), then strain out the water and keep the nuts in the fridge. They are nice and crunchy this way, and not soggy.

Unsoaked nuts contains enzyme inhibitors that make it harder to digest their fat. These inhibitors are part of a seed's self-preservation. They help keep a seed dormant while it's dry. That's also why you soak some seeks for a bit before planting to "wake them up." Once a nut is soaked, it's "awake" rather than dormant, and it is a lot easier for you to digest.

The fat that you get from an avocado comes in fatty acid form, which is easier to digest than fat itself. Nut-fat is not in fatty acid form, but when nuts are soaked they don't make you feel sick or heavy. You don't get fat eating nuts that are soaked, or avocadoes. Unlike eating butter or cheese, you don't get fat eating coconut oil. Coconut oil is a natural source of medium-chain tryglycerides (MCTs), which are quickly absorbed by your cells. This means coconut oil is not easily stored by your body as fat because your body prefers to use it up. If you eat this slow-burning fuel, you can go longer between meals. In fact, I have known some people who lost quite a bit of weight when they started eating coconut oil as their primary fat source (not more than 2-4 tablespoons per day).

Coconut oil has gotten flack as a saturated fat, but it is actually an excellent fat source. Not only is good fat useful as fuel, but eating good fat makes it easier for your body to make vitamins, deliver vitamins, and engage in many other chemical reactions. Fried chicken is not good fat. In fact, the more your fat gets cooked, the longer the fat molecule is, and the more work it takes for your body to get it ready for use. Sometimes fat molecules are so complex we can't use them correctly or at all, such as the trans-fats or hydrogenated fats in processed food, fast food, prepackaged baked goods and so on. In this condition, the fat molecule is similar to a molecule of plastic.

During my period of insomnia, I developed great sensitivity to any food containing corn products, soybean oil, canola oil, and soy sauce. After eating something with any of these ingredients, I would be tipsy as though I was mildly drunk, for a couple days afterward. These foods are genetically modified, and whatever they did to my gut bacteria made me feel drunk while trying to digest them. Now that I'm sleeping, if I'm in a situation where I can't avoid these ingredients, at least I'm not sick for a couple days afterward. This is just one example of an insomniac's compromised functioning. Cut out canola, soy and corn products as much as you can. Also, cut out foods with dyes, artificial and "natural" flavors, and MSG (monosodium glutamate). MSG makes us secrete a lot more insulin than normal and essentially makes us fat. It's also a neurotoxin that makes us addicted to the foods it's in. MSG has many names now--watch out for it as natural flavor, malt flavoring, yeast extract, glutamic acid, glutamate, or any food ingredient listed as hydrolized, protein-fortified, ultra-pasteurized and enzyme-modified.[24] Yes, those big food companies are very sneaky, and they don't care if you and your children get sick or sterile.

When you are trying to fix your insomnia, it's also a good idea to eat lightly and simply so you conserve some of your limited energy for activities other than digesting. Humans spend quite a bit of energy digesting food. When you eat less, the physical toll of getting nutrients out of your food, and then getting the waste products out of your body, is significantly reduced. Eating heavy meals makes an insomniac really exhausted, and saps what tiny bit of strength you have left. Don't eat after supper; keep your stomach empty so you can get the benefits of deep sleep, like making growth hormone and happy brain chemicals. Think about how turbulent your sleep is sometimes after a big heavy meal; you might have a lot of weird dreams, and toss and turn. You might feel rough or sluggish until you finally poop that meal out.

Eating lightly and simply has the additional benefit of reducing your total sleep time, also. When you eat less, you need less sleep. For example, when I do a short water fast (about one week without food, and drinking only water) I usually sleep about three or four hours per night without needing a nap during the day. I do this a couple times a year to clean out. During Christmas season, when my mom's yummy Italian cooking sucks me into total gluttony and I drink half a liter of vino a night, I spend about eight or nine fitful hours per night in bed, and generally feel quite sluggish during the days and not very well rested.

In the fourth year into my five years of severe insomnia, I developed terrible abdominal pain. A trip to the emergency and lots of tests revealed a benign tumor in my liver the size of a grapefruit. It was extremely painful; I was no longer able to lie down in horizontally to rest, drive a car, or even inhale comfortably. Coincidentally, by this time, I had also developed compulsive hunger and a thyroid problem. I craved fat, and would actually eat a few teaspoons of butter on its

---

[24] Erb, John and Michelle, The Slow Poisoning of America (Palladins Press, 2003).

own every day, in addition to lots of ice cream, sausage and chocolate. I gained twenty-five pounds *after* my second son's birth, in about six months, from my compulsive eating. I never felt satiated and I couldn't stop thinking about eating.

Since the liver problem was so excruciatingly painful, and the doctors had no idea how to handle the pain in the short-term, I had to do something on my own. I had to do it quickly. I did a few liver cleanses and passed *thousands* of green and yellow stones, many of which were calcified (yellow, hard and crusty instead of green and goopy). Some of the big yellow crusty ones were about an inch long! I decided to do a long water fast since this was the only way I knew to create rapid body change. I went 17 days on water only, without eating, and lost about 35 pounds. The critical pain went away, and a subsequent MRI revealed the tumor to be dissolved. I can only assume my liver's ability to do its job was compromised from the constant fatty food, the stones and the big-ass tumor.

This might explain why, when my heart would start racing at bedtime, I wouldn't be able to sleep all night long; I just simply didn't have the ability to get rid of the adrenaline. Even now, if I have a bad fight with my family before bed, I may not fall asleep at all, even though I can remain sort of calm and practice Banish / Gratitude repeatedly. Needless to say, I don't *ever* choose to have difficult conversations in the evening! I back away from any provocation simply in order to protect my night's sleep.

After the water fast, I went on diet of uncooked fruits and vegetables only, and the improvement in my mood and energy was incredible and immediate.[25] The fast fixed the racing heart problem at night. I was no longer consumed with anger. I was much calmer, and my resting heart rate went down to about 70-80 beats per minute. Even though I'd still be awake quite a bit during the night, I found it much easier to stay calm and I'd feel pretty good the next day with just a few hours sleep. I had much more physical stamina during the days.

While I'm not recommending anything extreme like a water fast, I want to emphasize the results of my experiment: if you eat less, and if what you eat is light and unprocessed, you will have more energy, you will feel more relaxed, you will find it easier to rest calmly when you're

---

[25] Victoria Boutenko's numerous books, videos and newsletters are an excellent source for learning how to add more fruit and vegetables to your diet. www.rawfamily.com.

awake, and you'll need to spend less time in bed. Your diet needs to be clean and light to help you make happy chemicals and minimize the effort your body requires to digest, process and detoxify.

To replace the flavor of processed foods and keep your palette satisfied, use garlic, onion, cayenne, turmeric, basil, oregano, dulse, lemon, and honey. Conveniently, many of these are thought to have strong liver cleansing properties, and the cleaner your liver is, the faster you will process your stress hormones. Some of these, like the acid of a lemon or garlic, will cleanse your liver by binding with, for example, some pesticides, and then you can eliminate the toxin normally, through urine, feces, and sweat. Otherwise it stays stuck in your liver and tissues.

It's possible that one reason insomnia keeps you raging with anger and paranoia is due to your reduced ability to get rid of your toxins and stress hormones. I felt terribly, uncontrollably angry all the time when I was in the insomnia abyss, and now I'm pretty calm most of the time.

In my experience, when the burden of digestion is removed, you feel much calmer even though you are not sleeping more. It makes it a lot easier to get from moment to moment without a meltdown or breakdown. I can't overstate the importance of general calmness. Once you are no longer at the whim of your toxic thoughts and stress hormones, you start to spiral up and up. The calmer you are, the faster you doze off. The less likely you are to jerk awake with a pounding heart after your first sleep cycle. The easier it becomes to control your thoughts. The easier it gets to invoke peaceful thoughts. Once you are pointed in the "up" direction, you are now teaching yourself to sleep again. You are practicing the art of sleeping, and as with all disciplines, the more you practice the better and easier it gets and the better you feel.

My heart happened to stop its night-time racing during my seventeen days of water fasting. I feel confident that I could have achieved this with the unprocessed diet and the practice of Banish / Gratitude at night, but the water fast compressed the practice period. I have always done my water fasts unsupervised, but there are many excellent clinics to help you should you wish some guidance.[26]

---

[26] Tanglewood Wellness Center (www.tanglewoodwellnesscenter.com), True North (www.healthpromoting.com); Tree of Life (www.gabrielcousens.com), The Koyfman Center (www.kofymancenter.com), and many more. These are just the organizations that I've been in touch with personally, and who have taken the

Western cultures aren't very familiar with water fasting, but Asians and Russians routinely practice water fasting for health reasons. It's not so difficult once you've done it a couple times, and the health benefits are extraordinary and immediate. Although it seems hard, it's actually a lot more effective than pharmaceuticals, and it's a lot better than percolating in your disease and discomfort. However, if you're a person with food addiction issues, I don't recommend a water fast, as it might make your psychological attachment worse, and start a yo-yo weight-gain-loss problem.

You can achieve the same amazing results just by cutting out processed food and sugary food. You can still stuff your face and feel satisfied. Instead of pasta, rice, and bread, eat a potato or yam. Yams are also delicious uncooked. For a sweet fix, have a bit of nice chocolate, fruits, or poach an apple or pear and mix with cinnamon; this really yummy! When I need a sweet fix, I like to mix a bit of honey with coconut oil, add a drop of peppermint flavor, harden it in the fridge, and voila, you have peppermint fudge. There are many diet practices you can follow, such as the Candida diet, where you can have delicious, balanced meals that are easy to prepare and filling.[27] Just be moderate with the nuts and fat!

Oh, in case I hadn't mentioned it…when you are not eating processed or sugary foods, you are going to lose weight. Even if you're full all the time. It is guaranteed. So give it a shot!

Supplements, Superfoods, and Natural Sleeping Aids

There are a number of dietary supplements you can try to help ensure you're getting the right minerals and vitamins for your body's laboratory to do its best chemical work. Unfortunately industrial agricultural practices deplete the soil of nutrients, so even the unprocessed food we eat now is of less benefit to us than it was thirty years ago. I require a double-dosage of vitamin D to ride through the Calgary winter, even though it is very sunny here. Magnesium is a mineral which serves a host of useful functions and is worth supplementing. I feel more relaxed when I take a magnesium

---

time to answer my questions about fasting. There are also numerous prestigious clinics in Russia and the Ukraine that will be less expensive but just as good if not better.

[27] Terry Willard of the Wild Rose College is one of the Candida diet pioneers and has published a recipe book that is easy and quick to follow. http://www.wrc.net.

supplement. My mother noticed a same-day reduction in the amount of ankle-swelling and foot pain she experiences. I also eat a bit of organic seaweed and put a bit of organic powdered kelp in my smoothie to get other trace minerals, like iodine. You use very little of these, so they are not expensive.

Many of the superfoods that are popular today, like maca power, cacao nibs, and acai nibs make me jittery. Insomniacs should avoid these. What about yerba maté? Stay away from this caffeinated plant; it gives me a worse buzz than coffee. I did and still do enjoy a cup of chamomile or sleepy-time tea. During my time in crisis, I found relaxing teas to be, well, relaxing. This may be from the ritual of the tea, the warmth, as well as the impact of the herbs.

What about natural sleeping aids? I tried a melatonin supplement, and found that it helped with sleep onset for a couple days (That it, it made me sleepy at bed time). But, after a couple days I noticed no effect. However, I know some people who have taken melatonin for years and swear by it; one pill before going to bed, and another when they awaken in the middle of the night.

I had a similar reaction to valerian; it made me sleepy at bedtime for a couple days, but didn't help me get into deep sleep or stay asleep, and soon thereafter I didn't notice the effect at all.

I also tried a natural sleeping aid called 5-HTP, which is the naturally occurring amino acid oxitriptan. This amino acid is needed by your body when you make serotonin and melatonin from tryptophan. I only tried it for one night and it made me so buzzed I didn't even fall asleep. I don't recommend this as a sleeping aid.

Exercise

Exercise plays a role in improving your sleep. It helps you process your food and toxins faster. It generates happy chemicals like endorphins. It metabolizes (uses up) your stress hormones, and improves your circulation. The insomniac needs some physical activity every day, preferably a few times a day for a short period. It doesn't have to be hard. You may not have the stamina and strength to push yourself during hard exercise. At my worst I could barely walk up a hill, let alone go for a long run.

Everyone has a different favorite exercise, something that makes you feel really good and that you enjoy. The "fun" aspect is very important: if you do something you don't enjoy, you won't make as many happy chemicals. I'm not a very physical or athletic person, but I do enjoy weight lifting, yoga and walking. I don't do a lot of it, but I do at least something once a day, either an exercise DVD, some squats or benchpress in the basement, or a walk outside. I've got a few of Jillian Michael's exercise DVD's. They are challenging and short, and inexpensive. Her attitude cracks me up, and she makes it fun. The programs are all suitable for beginners as well as more athletic people. If you can't do the exercises at first, she shows you a beginner modification you can work with instead.

Walking barefoot on grass or sand, walking in a forest, walking near water (like an ocean, river, or pond), dance, and yoga have the most powerful "reboot" effect on me. I found Bikram yoga (in a hot and humid yoga studio) very effective at dissipating anger and anxiety quickly, and for increasing clarity. But I didn't have time to attend a 90 minute exercise session away from my kids, and I didn't have the strength to get through such a long session without fainting. I would compress the sequence into a twenty or thirty minute series of poses in the family room after the kids were asleep. It was refreshing, calming and centering. I'd have a favorite television show and do the poses, so it didn't feel like "exercise."

However, once I was sleeping a few hours in a row each day, I did attend two real classes in a yoga studio and found them to be amazing. They were uplifting, challenging and motivating. If you can commit to something like this at least once a week, you will experience remarkable results. If you find the Bikram poses too challenging, try a basic sun salutation, which is shorter but still very beneficial, can be done anywhere, and for free. For women with back problems, both lower and upper, the usefulness of yoga cannot be overstated. Yoga is something that's better to learn in a class or watching a video, rather than from a book, so make the investment in some training. Every public library has plenty of yoga DVDs, and Jillian Michaels also has a yoga DVD, which I bought for a whopping seven dollars at Wal-Mart.

For the insomniac, the supreme value of your exercise lies in its effectiveness at helping you make happy chemicals, not in how hard it is or how skinny it will make you. You may need to lay off some hard exercise to help yourself recover. People who train too hard put a strain on their systems. For example, men who work out too frequently don't get the necessary recovery time and hence they start making less testosterone. Runners who push themselves too hard before a race tend to have depressed immune systems and are more vulnerable to catching colds and flu's.

Against my natural workaholic tendencies, I've recently committed to a weekly Zumba class, and I love it! I can push myself a lot harder in the class than I do on my own, and even though I'm not very coordinated or quick, I still enjoy learning and trying the choreography.[28] I feel a great lightness of being and natural buzz after the class, much more so than when I run. This has to do with the type of exercise. When you move your arms a lot, high above the head, you stimulate what's called lymph drainage. Sedentary people (most of us who work at a desk) don't move and drain our lymph system enough.

Your lymph system contains a lot more liquid than you have blood in your body, but unlike the blood which has its own pump (the heart), lymph juice gets moved around when we contract our muscles in certain ways, like during Tai-Chi's long, flowing movements, or when conducting an orchestra. Mini-trampolines, also called Rebounders, are supposed to be effective at moving lymph juice around. To move your lymph fluids around, you don't need to do something taxing on the cardiovascular system like running. You just need to move around.

When I lived in San Francisco, I saw a lot of elderly Asians bouncing gently in place in Washington square, their heads, jaws and arms relaxed, loose and flopping slightly. I learned this is called "ching-ing" and it stimulates the lymph drainage. This is one reason you feel really good when dancing or engaging in a sport where you get to move more freely and play like a child.

Exercise basics: as you know, don't do any hard exercise shortly before bedtime, or you won't be able to fall asleep. Save your harder exercise for at least 4-8 hours before you retire. But if you don't have any other time for exercise, then do something more relaxing like yoga or chinging close to bedtime. If you get really twitchy in the night, some yoga and stretching can help get rid of the jitters by using up some of your stress hormones.

The weight loss from the water fast made me look and feel a lot better. I hate to sound shallow and vain, but I am a bottom-heavy woman and was really happy to be back into size six pants. For the first time after having kids, when I looked into the mirror, I felt surprise and delight rather than disgust and shame. The effects of good diet and exercise are on your self-esteem are profound, and the

---

[28] My instructor is an amazing Hungarian hot mama named Bogi Gergely, http://boglarka3.zumba.com.

satisfaction makes your happy hormones kick into gear. That's why you feel relaxed when you accomplish something. You feel gratitude and pride in your efforts. The cycle spins up and up from there. You take more care with what goes in and are less likely to commit random acts of self-sabotage. You have just a little more peace of mind, and so you sleep a bit better.

As well, after losing weight, and getting a bit stronger from exercise, I wasn't uncomfortable in my bed all the time. I had tried several mattresses during my years as an insomniac, but could never seem to get comfortable. Soft mattress, hard mattress, magnetic mattress, futons of varying density and thickness, memory foam. I'd have a pillow between my knees, or one under my ankle and two under my knees and one under each elbow, and I'd be readjusting all this stuff all night long.

During my first pregnancy I developed severe sciatica, and this never seemed to go away completely. When I was heavier, my lower back and hips ached constantly, and so did my ankles and feet. I started growing cankles. The pain prevented me from sleeping as deeply, because it was uncomfortable to stay in one spot for very long, and every shift required effort. When I lost some weight, the back and foot pain disappeared, and so did the swelling in my ankles. I might have been able to handle the pain and extra weight a bit more easily had I been sleeping well and my systems working better. Without sleep, the pain and extra weight posed extra problems for my compromised abilities. Losing some weight makes you happier and more comfortable and will make it easier to sleep.

Get Outside

For all humans, the benefits of being out in nature cannot be overstated. It's our own personal reboot button. The fresh air, the sunlight, and the earth's electrical field have great benefit for us in ways that haven't yet been quantified by science. Spending time in nature is something we overlook frequently. Take a walk after supper or play with your kids outside. Commit to doing some exercise in some green space or near some water at least a couple times a week. Go splash in some shallow water. Get out and watch the sunrise, or the sunset and stars at night. Reconnect yourself to the phases of the moon; catch a moonrise or moonset. I like to lie on my back on the grass or even in the snow and watch the night sky occasionally. It doesn't have to be for a long time; just a few minutes. Reconnecting to the earth, moon and stars can have the effect of pulling you out of your bubble of complaints.

Recent research shows that taking a morning walk in the sunlight can help you reset your body clock to match up with our natural circadian rhythms. This is because the part of our brain that regulates the sleep-wake cycle is close to the nerve that links our eyes to our brains. Scientists now know that light makes us happy, alert and trains our body clocks, but too much bright light at night signals our clocks to delay.

Sex

No discussion of exercise could be complete without a referral to the oldest exercise of all, next to gathering food: sex! Sex, practiced with love and affection, is a great way to generate happy hormones and endorphins. Studies show that couples with regular sex live longer with less disease. During my period as an insomniac, I lost all interest in sex, but when my husband actually managed to convince me to get naked, I always felt better afterward. Even if you're not interested in sex, it will still benefit you, so make some time for it, and surprise yourself with how fun it is!

#4: Adjust your Environment and Habits

Some small changes in environment and habit will also make a difference in your overall peacefulness and help improve your sleep:

Sync With Your Internal Clock

Go to bed earlier so you sync up better with your internal clock. Our cortisol levels are naturally at their lowest a few hours after going to bed, and you get more deep sleep in the early part of the night, so if you can commit to getting to bed around ten in the evening, you are more likely to have more deep sleep. I know this seems early, but it doesn't have to be forever, only while you are trying to sort out your medical emergency. Take a walk after supper instead of flopping on to the sofa; this will help you digest before bedtime, and lower your insulin levels. If you do watch TV, dim the lights and don't sit too close.

Try to get to bed about the same time each night, and if you need to get up early to go to work, cut out some evening activities so you can spend at least seven or eight hours in bed. We stay up late to get more done, but in the long run this is harmful to our health. Make this investment while you're trying to restore sleep health; you're worth it. The dirty floor and those emails or projects can wait.

Keep your bedroom clean, uncluttered and cozy, and free of electrical devices like television, tablet, computer, cell phone, cordless phone and fluorescent lights. The tidiness and comfort of your sleeping area affects your subconscious mind, and helps you relax more easily. Make sure your mattress, pillows, sheets and blankets are comfortable and clean. Don't drink too much fluid at night, so you won't have to get up and pee and risk not falling back asleep. Oh yeah, sex before bed can help you sleep better, too!

Television is too stimulating before bed; don't watch it for at least an hour before retiring. The way it makes color and images is stimulating for your brain in a way that we're not conscious of. Also, it's full of messages that tell you're not good enough unless you have whiter teeth, a smaller butt, a new big car, and so on. Avoid working on your computer before bedtime; its brightness will interfere with your melatonin clock. For example, most of this book was written at night after I put my kids to bed, so between 9pm and 1am. That gave me five hours for sleep, which for me is a decent amount, but I found it hard to fall asleep and I slept very lightly and feel quite tired now that I'm nearly done.

Don't do anything too stimulating before bed, like engage in a fight with your spouse or kids. Walk away from any battle, for you are now a soldier for sleep and nothing else. Picking up your iPhone or iPad in the middle of the night if you can't sleep is very tempting, so keep them out of the bedroom also. If you want to do something in the middle of the night, like read or listen to some relaxing music, make a habit of leaving your bed to do it. I've known some people who found this practice very helpful, for they decided that it was too much work to get out of the bed, and so they just stayed in the bed and eventually nodded off. If you're really twitchy in the night, try some simple yoga poses; they help you dissipate stress hormones much more quickly than regular stretching.

If you must have a phone in your bedroom, use a land line phone that is not cordless. Our devices, particularly our wireless ones, have emissions that can impact our sleep negatively. To help block out light, use heavy drapes or black-out curtains. A quick fix that's inexpensive is to buy a couple yards of black-out material or heavy, dark fabric and velcro it to your curtains.

If your bedroom is too noisy, you need to find another room in your house or apartment for sleeping. Anything that bothers you becomes the sole focus of your concentration when you're up in the middle of the night. I frequently sleep with construction headphones on, as earplugs don't give me enough relief from the street traffic. They weren't comfortable at first, and my ears don't like being plugged up and sweaty after a while, but that's what it took to block out the noise. I never travel without them now! If you wear the headphones over a hoodie, then your ears don't get so sweaty.

Under the construction headphones I'd have my listening headphones on, playing classical music, favorite mellow news programs (not inflammatory shock-jock style--that's a no-no at night!) or a guided meditation. Some people recommend a "white noise" machine. I find it annoying, but the white noise machine used to be the only way we could get my oldest to sleep more than thirty minutes at a time!

A bath before bed with candles and lavender oil? Yep. This is a lot better than television. Just don't count on this alone to restore your healthy sleep habits. A long but not too long (thirty minutes) warm bath will relax your muscles. Keep the lighting low to stimulate melatonin production, so try candles and relaxing music. Stretch. Meditate or pray. Read. Sauna. Chamomile tea. Write in your journal. Anything except playing with your electronic devices or watching television right before bed. A relaxing ritual that you believe in, that you create just for you, and that you enjoy, is going to help you wind down for sleeping.

Gadgets

During my insomniac years, I became very sensitive to electrical frequencies. I do not understand exactly how or why this is, but it has something to do with how compromised all your functions are when you are chronically sleep deprived. Even now, I still cannot use wireless internet for very long and I rarely use a cordless phone, let alone a cell phone up next to my head; these devices make me nauseous within about ten minutes. Apparently about ten percent of the population has a hard time tolerating electro-magnetic frequencies (EMF). In my experience, when you are not sleeping enough, your sensitivity to EMF increases. This is another reason to keep your electrical devices out of your bedroom. Even if you think this is hocus-pocus, try it anyway. Just because you're not aware of the effect of EMF on you at night doesn't mean it's not happening, and every small thing matters when you are solving a medical emergency.

It is through my increased sensitivity to EMF that I learned why walking barefoot in sand or in and near bodies of water makes you feel good. It's an electrical matter. We build up a surplus of positive ions, and the beach or bodies of water have a surplus of negative ions. Like lightning, we discharge our positive charge to the negative ground (minus the large bolt of static electricity). This happens without our knowing. What we do know is that we feel better outside. Part of curing your own insomnia is learning to trust your feelings and intuition. It's important to go with your flow, and not to fight your nature. If it feels better, it will help you relax and make fewer stress hormones, no questions asked!

One theory about our increased sensitivity to EMF has to do with chem-trails, which refers to the widespread aerial (i.e., from airplanes) spraying of chemicals, such as barium, aluminum and silver solutions, for a variety of covert purposes, such as adjusting local weather patterns to prevent big hailstones from forming. With more metal in the air and on the ground, we are more conductive than we used to be.

Grounding Sheet

Thanks to my gadget-happy husband I tried what's called a "grounding sheet", which is supposed to reduce the impact of EMF at night by connecting you to the earth's electrical field. There is some dispute about how these work and how effective they are. During my period of insomnia, I noticed that it was getting harder to use a cell phone or cordless phone, or even stand near a working microwave or photocopier. My bed is about twenty yards from a large transformer, and hence we thought to try the grounding sheet.

I noticed the difference immediately, and for me the effect was very relaxing. I was able to achieve deep relaxation very quickly, and reach deep sleep. Upon waking, even in the middle of the night, I remained in a fuzzy relaxed state without the racing heart.

The theory behind the grounding or "earthing" sheet goes like this: the earth has an electric field (free electrons) that we are also able to conduct unless we're wearing plastic or rubber shoes, or stuck in a wood or plastic house or office. You feel it as peaceful tingling when you're out walking barefoot near the water on a beach, on a stretch of wet grass, or in a forest. You might not notice any physical change, but you will notice your improved mood. Since the earth's field is continuous direct current, the 60Hz alternating current systems we use in our homes and workplaces are not natural for us. The grounding sheet is conductive and is supposed to transfer the free electrons of the earth's field to your body. The sheet is woven through with wires, and you plug it into the grounding input of an electrical socket (the fat one on the bottom).[29]

My husband also tried sleeping on the sheet, but did not notice any impact, whereas I was even able to feel whether or not the sheet was plugged in. The grounding sheet's claim to fame comes from a doctor's experiment with a winning American Tour de France cycling team. With the grounding sheets during sleep, the athletes' cortisol levels normalized and synchronized with our body circadian or natural clock, which has cortisol at its lowest level about midnight. As you now know, lower nighttime cortisol levels result in deeper sleep and the production / release of happy chemicals that keep your mind and body working optimally.

I found that I couldn't't use the sheet long term. A couple weeks on, then a couple weeks off. My mother uses the grounding sheet and finds it helpful for the swelling in her ankles, but doesn't notice the difference for sleeping. My father tried it but didn't notice the difference for sleeping, and he thinks we're all crazy anyway. However, my mother thinks he snores less when sleeping on the sheet.

Magnetic Therapy

I also experimented with magnetic therapy, which is supposed to improve circulation, provide pain relief, and promote relaxation. My husband built a magnetic base for our mattress using about 700 pounds of commercial magnets lined up on a plywood base onto which we plopped our Ikea memory foam futon. The difference between the grounding sheet and magnetic therapy is that magnets don't provide the free electrons and the balancing effect of the earth's electrical frequencies. I didn't notice that the magnetic helped or

---

[29] The principal retailer of grounding products is a company named Earthing. (www.earthing.com). They also retail via Upaya Naturals (www.upayanaturals.com).

interfered with sleeping. However, I did notice some impact on relaxation, just not as powerful an effect as the grounding sheet. Its most powerful effect came when I sprained my thumb. I wrapped a small magnet under a tensor bandage and slept with this on. That little magnet wrapped onto my thumb spent the whole night trying to get to its big magnet friends underneath me; it throbbed against my thumb all night long. When I got up in the morning I had a magnet-shaped dark bruise on my thumb pad from all this effort. Remarkably, I had almost full range of motion restored! It was the fastest I'd ever healed a sprained thumb. Normally I can't play the piano for at least a month after twisting my thumb back the wrong way.

Some say magnets increase blood flow to the area they touch by attracting the iron in the blood and by relaxing capillary walls, the surrounding muscle and the connective tissue. The increased blood flow brings more oxygen and nutrients to the injured or painful body part, thus speeding up the healing process. Others say that iron is bound to hemoglobin inside our blood cells and consequently cannot be affected by the presence of any magnetic field produced by a commercial magnet. While there aren't any negative side effects, magnetic therapy is not for anyone with an electro-medical device like a pacemaker, nor for pregnant women and infants.

Air Filters

As my insomnia worsened, I became increasingly sensitive to odors and dust. I got nauseous at the smell of shampoo and toothpaste, and wasn't able to use common household cleaning products. If the air seemed dusty at night while I was lying awake, trying to sleep, I would fixate on it; it would drive me bonkers and bingo, my heart would start racing as I launched fight-flight. To help with this, we purchased air filters and purifiers and an ozone machine to keep the air in our home cleaner. If you live or work in a new building, the off-gassing of all the plastic materials used in construction may be interfering with your sleep. For some reason, our small house is older, not very well insulated, and happens to be very dusty. We are on a corner lot facing northwest near a large open area. We don't have any trees, so we may be collecting a lot of dust from the outside, or it could be our old wall-to-wall carpeting. In my insomnia-induced hypersensitivity, I frequently found the air quality bothersome when trying to fall asleep. The air-cleaning machines were worthwhile for me, and they are not expensive. The air purifiers were $70, and the ozone machine about $100. My methodical husband also vacuums every day and measures the dust we generate. We change our furnace filter every few months.

Sauna

In addition to keeping us cool, perspiration serves the very important function of cleaning our bodies. Our bodies eliminate most toxins naturally by sweating. I happen to be one of those weirdoes who doesn't break a sweat, even with hard exercise. I'll get as red as a tomato climbing out of the Grand Canyon on a summer day, but nary a drop of perspiration to be found. When my liver tumor was diagnosed, I knew I needed some way to support my sick liver in cleaning out my body. My husband decided it was time to figure out how to sweat, so he bought an infrared sauna. An infrared sauna doesn't need the complex plumbing of a stream room, and warms you up without getting the sauna itself really hot. It's basically easier and less expensive to have this type of sauna than a steam room or traditional dry sauna. Infrared heat warms objects only in its direct path and has a lesser effect on the temperature of the surrounding air. It's like when you're outside in the summer, feeling hot, but then you feel cool when a cloud blocks out the sun. The temperature of the air has not changed, but you are receiving less of the sun's infrared rays. These aren't harmful; they're not like a microwave, and they don't age you prematurely like ultraviolet rays. But you get really hot. When you're in a sauna, your heart works harder to pump blood to support increased sweat production. The heat simply speeds up the body's natural process of cleaning out toxins through the skin. What comes out through your skin? Toxins such as sodium, alcohol, nicotine, cholesterol carcinogenic heavy metals (like cadmium, lead, zinc, nickel), and a lot more.[30]

The first time I used the sauna for fifteen minutes, I overheated and fainted. The next day I think I found a bead or two of sweat. Within a couple weeks I was sweating profusely in about twenty minutes, even soaking the towel I was sitting on. I'd usually lose about half a pound in the sauna in about 40 minutes. It's easy to stay in

[30] Dr. Toshiko Yamazaki, M.D., owns a clinic in Japan where she has done extensive research on the therapeutic uses of far infrared. Her books is The Science of Far-Infrared Therapies.

there. Since the sauna itself doesn't get very warm, I put my laptop on the floor and watch a show or read a magazine. An infrared sauna costs about $500 for a single-person sauna. Ours is a 4-person sauna (four very little people!) and was $3000. We've been using the same sauna now at least four times per week for four years, so it has more than paid off our initial investment.

The main benefit of heat and perspiration for the insomniac? After taking a sauna before bed I was so relaxed I was able to fall asleep in less than an hour, and stay asleep sometimes for four hours in a row. It was the first time in a decade that I'd ever slept four hours in a row. It felt like a miracle. Also, after a sauna, I woke up after three or four hours feeling deeply rested.

Listening Materials

But after three hours of sleep, then what? After this much sleep, I was unlikely to fall asleep again. If I did, I might just doze lightly, but not feel like I was resting deeply. The key to riding this time until you're sleeping more hours in a row is to enjoy yourself at night when you're awake. For me, it was Banish/Gratitude and listening to guided meditations and helpful listening material, as well as favorite music. In particular, I enjoyed Mozart. It's orderly, beautiful, filled with love and harmony and hope. If you Banish / Gratitude while listening to a piece of music, you can condition your reflexes just like Pavlov's dog. Even now, three years later, I still experience a surge of euphoria when I hear the finale of the Marriage of Figaro, because I spent so many hours associating it with the expression of gratitude during my night-time listening.

It is said that there are many levels of consciousness between alertness and deep sleep. During my time in the insomnia abyss, I'd frequently be lucid-sleeping and lucid-dreaming. I have since lost these abilities, which is too bad, because it was actually quite interesting and enjoyable. I was able to hear noises around me; I was aware that I was not in deep sleep nor awake, and also aware that I couldn't move. At some level I could feel that body restoration was in progress and that my body was not going to let me interrupt it. The sensation was similar to sailing on a very smooth ocean. Sometimes I could even move out of my body and leave the house, right through the walls or roof. This may have been a dream, but it was frequent and seemed real, because I felt alert and remember it so clearly, moving around in the darkness and watching the sky and stars.

I also engaged in lucid dreaming, where I was conscious of dreaming. I was frequently able to direct the dream. Both of these activities brought me a sense of great ease and enjoyment, like having my own private holodeck. Alas, I didn't have many hot sex dreams, but I did have a lot of action-adventure Indiana-Jones-style dreams, where there was an exciting quest and stimulating historical context. Instead of running on the spot when being chased by a bad guy, I was aware that I was dreaming and could do whatever I wanted, so I'd start flying or taking large leaps. It felt very freeing to be in control and alert. I knew I was having fun and was careful not to come out of the dream.

I also experienced what I believe to be vague premonition dreams; for example, in the months before the Fukishima nuclear accident in 2011, I had dozens of tsunami nightmares. These were pretty scary, but also interesting, because I knew my mind was beginning to transcend normal physical limitations of time and space.

The bottom line is that for insomniacs, even when you're not sleeping, you can be in an in-between state that is restorative. You can be lucid but aware that you're still allowing body-repair. It might not be slow-wave sleep, but it's a lot better than being angry and frustrated. For me, I think the main benefit of these states was the fun I had. It was the first time in many years that I had associated sleep with something enjoyable. Instead of dreading the long hours awake, I began to look forward to the night's secret adventures, and appreciate the fact that I'd remember everything and could write it down. Why was this good? By now you should know what I'm going to say: because I didn't start secreting stress hormones in the middle of the night!

If I was too tired or bored for Banish / Gratitude, I kept a variety of listening materials at the ready. Classical music, non-shock-jock news, or guided meditations. I keep my ancient Philips MP3 player at the bedside so I can easily find it in the dark without having to turn on the light or move around. I organize the folders so I can find the good night-time materials and music very quickly in the dark. This prevents me from having to think too much or get too alert. I have some favorite guided meditations and self-hypnosis tracks that I have listened to thousands of times in the middle of the night over the years. They are effective at helping you relax, and numerous repetitions create a conditioned relaxation reflex, so that after a while, all you have to do is start the playback and you descend into deep relaxation in less than a minute. It is important to find a voice and style you like. Some self-help gurus have abrasive speaking voices, or annoying phrasing and mannerisms that you will find very irritating in your hypersensitive nighttime state.

Self-hypnosis and guided meditations also have some other deeper effect that I like to call "cleaning out your subconscious." The practice of hypnosis teaches us that toxic thoughts can be released without conscious analysis. Most people may do their releasing during deep sleep and while dreaming, but if you are like me, you may have gone years without sleeping long enough to dream and don't have the opportunity to clean your mind out in this way. Self-hypnosis facilitates the cleaning without the deep or dream sleep.

I didn't have any interest in self-hypnosis or hypnosis before getting desperate for answers. While I don't doubt that governments engage in Manchurian Candidate manipulation, the kind of self-hypnosis and hypnosis you undertake to help with insomnia is nothing like you see at county fairs, where people do and say silly things without any memory afterward. In addition to my listening materials, I had six sessions with a private hypnotherapist, and found them to be helpful[31]. Physically, the extent of the hypnosis was not a "going under" but a deep relaxation that I had never known before while awake. For an hour after my session, my hands and legs felt too heavy and slow, but there was no irritation or frustration with it. Traffic, speech, and my own movements appeared to have slowed down. I was extremely calm and clear for about five hours after each session, and I was able to recall this sensation during the nights when I lay awake. This might be the chemical response that sleeping aids are aiming for, but hypnosis achieves it much more precisely and powerfully, minus the next-day fog and anxiety.

When I wasn't sleeping at all, I didn't have the ability to focus in order to practice meditation. The guided listening materials were really crucial to helping me stay calm at night. It took two years to get to the point where I could lie awake all night, still unable to sleep, but calm and accepting. When you're suffering from insomnia, everything becomes dark and filled with despair. It takes some time to retrain yourself to experience joy in life again. The guided listening materials provide a positive and pleasant alternative to your own angry voice cycling through your head.

---

[31] Maude Schelhous of Sacramento Hypnotherapy was my hypnotherapist (www.sacramentohypnotherapy.com).

Eventually I developed a meditation practice and a spiritual practice that is very meaningful to me now, but I wasn't capable of organizing my thoughts and intentions this way during my time of crisis. Personally, I don't know how helpful the traditional organized religions are for insomniacs. You can beg God to help you sleep but if you don't have a way to make happy chemicals and keep stress hormones at bay, you won't get very far, and you'll be angry that God isn't helping you sleep. A mindfulness practice that is self-responsible, rigorous and personal—like we are about physical exercise—will be of more immediate benefit. Or, you can pray and practice Banish / Gratitude; this is of great benefit also.

Many of the writers I've mentioned previously in this book are excellent sources of guided listening / meditation material. Deepak Chopra is an accessible place to start. I also listen to Doreen Virtue, Wayne Dyer, Marianne Williamson, Gary Renard and Jennifer Hadley. Most of these teachers offers hundreds of hours of free audio material and excellent online classes at a reasonable price. HayHouseRadio.com and Unity.fm are online radio stations that broadcast excellent spiritual / health programming 24/7 free of charge.

Patience

Restoring your sleep health is a habit that gets built up over time. The last thing I'd like to recommend is that you remember this and be patient with yourself. If you were recovering from a physical injury, you'd give yourself the time to heal, and it's the same with sleeping habits: you need some time to retrain your mind and restore your chemistry. There is no way you'll go from zero to five hours, or even from two hours to five hours overnight. My wish for you is that you will use this information here to journey out of the insomnia abyss faster than I did.

Summary

- Changes in attitude, lifestyle and habit are needed to solve your chemical problem by yourself. You are the boss, even if you don't feel like it or want to be!
- You must address both the physical component and the psychological component to get results.

Some actions you can take are listed below:

- Develop a mental practice of gratitude so you are calmer at night.
- Take appropriate action to handle your problems so they don't keep you awake at night.
- Get off drugs: sleeping aids, caffeine, alcohol, recreational drugs etc.
- Keep your diet light and unprocessed so that you maintain healthy blood sugar and conserve your energy for your body's healing work.
- Choose a fun exercise and do it regularly. Get outside.
- Make small changes in your environment and lifestyle so you sync up better with your internal clock.
- Listening to helpful or relaxing materials can help you enjoy this journey.
- Be patient, as you would have to be when recovering from a physical injury, like a broken ankle.

6 CONCLUSION

Today, nothing is more important than my efforts to sleep. I am too new to sleeping through the night and I don't take it for granted! I don't go out late at night very often, because I can't risk missing sleep and getting into a rut. I stopped travelling overseas because the jetlag is too stressful. I don't even travel much locally so that I won't interfere with my sleep schedule.

Don't get me wrong—I still have a pile of fun. But my fun has to be comprised of activities that don't conflict with my efforts to maintain healthy sleep, because I am too new to it. My life goal now is to be peaceful inside, and to cascade this into my little world. I'm not always successful. Any other objectives I hold are inconsequential if they disrupt my ability to be happy and peaceful.

Why? Because as soon as I'm agitated, my sleep suffers, and I never want to be in the insomnia abyss again. I was angry and miserable and wasn't any fun to be with. I am a busy type-A working mother, so it takes constant vigilance to prevent my driven personality from running the show, lest I descend into the insomnia abyss again. It takes constant mindfulness, as I miss the mark and readjust and correct. I now understand that constant mindfulness, constant self-correction and readjusting is normal and ok.

Thank you for taking the time to read this. I hope you find thoughts and suggestions here that are helpful for you. Above all, remember that you are not alone and you are not crazy. The sadness or despair you feel is shared by many insomniacs. The angry, bleak person you visit in the middle of your sleepless nights is not the true you. That's the sick you, even if it might feel like there is nothing else left of your personality.

You are the only one who can take control!

You can get your life back!

RESOURCES

BUYTEKO BREATHING METHOD

- Buteyko Breathing Organization
  http://buteykobreathing.org

- McKeon, Patrick, <u>Buteyko Clinic Method 2hr DVD, CD, Manual; the Complete Instruction to Reverse Asthma, Rhinitis and Snoring Permanently</u> (2008)

BOOKS & LISTENING MATERIALS

Most of these writers and teachers have dozens of excellent books available on audio; here I've just listed a few.

Wisdom Center Technologies

This is the best guided meditation I've ever listened to. I have listened to it thousands of times over the years ($21 + shipping). The music is terrific. Created and recorded by Jim DiGirolano, <u>Attunement for Life Series: Relax and Energize</u>.
   Available via http://www.californiainstitute.net/tape.htm

Jean Kowalski & Rosanna D'Agnillo

<u>Peaceful Journey</u>, Volumes 1 & 2 -
Available at www.rosannad.com
This two discs include a four meditation set (each is 30 minutes) with a different spiritual focus. The meditations were channeled by medium Jean Kowalski; I composed the music.

The Foundation for Inner Peace
www.acim.org

This is the organization that publishes <u>A Course in Miracles</u>. I consider this to be the most important book I've ever read. If you are ready to change your mind about everything, dive in and be amazed. Were I stuck on a desert island, this is the book I'd want with me.

Jennifer Hadley - www.jenniferhadley.com

Visit www.jenniferhadley.com to browse through her many classes available on CD and for download. Some are for sale, but she also provides, via iTunes, hundreds of free radio shows and classes. She also has a weekly radio show on Unity.FM. Please make a donation so Jennifer can continue to provide all of this awesome free material.

HayHouseRadio.com

You can join this network for a small annual fee of $48. It is well worth the money. This gives you download access to all of the excellent radio shows from many of America's greatest teachers of the mind-body connection, such as Dr. Wayne Dyer, Dr. Christiane Northrup, Caroline Myss, Doreen Virtue, and many others. You can also listen live and stream without paying the annual membership fee.

Unity.FM

This is the 24-hour online radio show broadcast for The Unity Online Radio Network, a "platform for spiritual and New Thought discussions. The programs on the network are a powerful voice in providing the consciousness, clarity and common vision necessary to create transformation in the world today." You can listen and download the radio shows without charge. Please make a donation if you can to help keep the station running.

Science Friday - http://sciencefriday.com/

I love science radio shows, since this is my only time to learn about the world of science, and the radio show makes it digestible. The topics are current and diverse, and the interviewers are intelligent and engaging. Science Friday is a weekly science radio show.

Quirks and Quarks - www.cbc.ca/quirks

This is a weekly Canadian science radio show, also very engaging.

Deepak Chopra

- <u>Stress Free with Deepak Chopra</u> (2011)
- <u>The Secret of Healing: Meditations for Transformation and Higher Consciousness</u> (2011).

- The Secret of Love: Meditations for Attracting and Being in Love (2011)
- The Soul of Healing Affirmations (2008)
- Chakra Balancing: Body, Mind and Soul (2004)
- The Soul of Healing Meditations (2001)

Gregg Easterbrook

- The Progress Paradox: How Life Gets Better While People Feel Worse (2004)
- Sonic Boom: Globalization at Mach Speed (2009)

John Gray

- Venus on Fire, Mars on Ice: Emotional Balance--The Key to Life, Love and Energy (2010)

Thich Nhat Hanh

- Peace is Every Step (1992)
- Peace is Every Breath (2011)

Esther Hicks/Abraham

- Getting Into The Vortex: Guided Meditations CD and User Guide (2010)
- The Teachings of Abraham: The Master Course CD Program, 11-CD set (2008)
- The Amazing Power of Deliberate Intent 4-CD (2006)

Gary Renard

- Fearless Love: The Answer to the Problem of Human Existence (2008)
- Your Immortal Reality (2007)
- Secrets of the Immortal: Advanced Teachings from A Course in Miracles (2006)
- The Disappearance of the Universe (2004)

Robert Schwartz

- Your Soul's Plan: Discovering the Real Meaning of the Life You Planned Before You Were Born (2010)
- Your Soul's Gift: The Healing Power of the Life You

<u>Planned Before You Were Born</u> (2012)

Colin Tipping
- <u>Radical Forgiveness: A Revolutionary Five-Stage Process to Heal Relationships, Let Go of Anger and Blame, Find Peace in Any Situation</u> (2009)

Brian Tracy
- <u>The Pscyhology of Achievement</u> (2002)

Doreen Virtue
- <u>Angel Therapy Meditations</u> (2008)
- <u>The Best of Doreen Virtue</u> (2006)
- <u>Angel Medicine</u> (2005)
- <u>Chakra Clearing</u> (2004)
- <u>Karma Releasing</u> (2004)
- <u>Manifesting with the Angels</u> (2003)

DIET RESOURCES
www.rawfamily.com
I have followed Victoria Boutenko for many years. She has a number of books and videos that teach you how to eat better. She is a big proponent of the "green smoothie", where you drink a smoothie with vegetables and fruits in it. It tastes like fruit, not the vegetables, so it's totally yummy and easy to drink.

www.juicefeasting.com
This is a 92 day juicing program developed by David and Katrina Rainoshek that has been profiled on mainstream television and has earned excellent results in causing the body to heal what ails it.

www.davidwolfe.com
David Wolfe is the original guru for a clean diet, and he's got a lot of great information for the novice. My only caveat would be that you don't need to buy the supplements to be healthy, and insomniacs should avoid the superfoods that give you the jitters, like maca, acai berries, and cacao nibs.

GROUNDING
Grounding products reduce the harmful effects of electromagnetic frequencies, and promote relaxation. They are available for sale directly at www.earthing.com. Also, many grounding products are sold by Upaya Naturals (www.upayanaturals.com).

HEALTH CENTERS/FASTING CLINICS
If you can afford it, the following institutions can help you bring about radical change in your sleeping and health. You can do these programs in your home, however; you don't have to pay someone else to help you eat and think better. There are many fasting clinics in the Ukraine and Russia also that provide hands-on medical supervision and cost less than the American facilities. The former Eastern bloc takes fasting seriously as a type of medical intervention, so the quality of the medical supervision is high.

Tree of Life Center
http://www.gabrielcousens.com/
(Patagonia, Arizona USA)
Run by Dr. Gabriel Cousens

Hippocrates Health Institute
http://www.hippocratesinst.org/
(West Palm Beach, Florida, USA)
Run by Drs. Brian and Anna Maria Clement

Here are some websites for fasting (water and "dry" fasting clinics in the former Soviet Union that are well-known and reputable.

http://filonov.net/
http://www.belovodie.com/
http://www.kohmaclinic.ru/prog/
http://centerrdt.com/
http://www.drdautov.ru/
http://lechebnoegolodanie.com/
http://www.revital.ru/
http://syhoegolodanie.com/

HYPNOTHERAPY

Maude Schellhous, Sacramento Hypnotherapy.
www.sacramentohypnotherapy.com. If you are outside of this area, they can help refer you to appropriate help.

WORKSHEETS & CHECKLISTS

Please visit my website at www.end-insomnia.com and www.rosannad.com to download free PDFs of any of the following worksheets and checklists in this book.

DAILY JOURNAL

When you are in crisis, it is useful to keep a journal so you can better and more accurately remember what is happening, and how you are caring for yourself. You may not need to use it for a long time, but even committing the time and effort to this puts your body and mind into active self-healing mode.

Seven things I am grateful for today:
1.
2.
3.
4.
5.
6.
7.

Issues and problems that I thought about instead of trying to sleep:
1.
2.
3.
4.

What can I do today to address those problems so that I can feel better tonight when it is time to sleep?
1.
2.
3.
4.

Time I fell asleep? _____

Time I hoped to wake up? _____

Time I actually got up in the morning? _____

How do I rate the quality of my sleep? _____

Any memorable dreams?

_____
_____
_____

How many times did I wake during the night; when & how long? What woke me up?

_____

_____

What I did when I was awake in the night?

_____

_____

_____

_____

How I felt today?

_____

_____

_____

_____

Did I nap today? For how long? How I felt after?

_____

_____

Did I exercise today? What did I do, and for how long?

_____

_____

_____

_____

What medications did I take today, and when?

_____

_____

Did I drink caffeine or alcohol or eat junk food? How much and when?

_____

_____

Here's what I ate today:

_____

_____

_____

_____

How do I rate my stress level, and what was I stressed about today?

_____

_____

_____

_____

What I did today to help generate happy hormones:

_____

_____

_____

_____

What I did in the two hours before retiring to bed?

_____

_____

_____

_____

What will I try differently today?

_____

_____

_____

_____

KNOW THYSELF....

What kind of self-soother are you? Assess how nervous and controlling a person you are:

_____

_____

_____

_____

Do you snore or experience sleep apnea?

_____

_____

_____

_____

How many years have you been sleeping poorly? Do you regularly feel tired or not refreshed even if you sleep for a long period?

_____

_____

_____

_____

What mix of circumstances and actions led up to it?

_____

_____

_____

_____

Is your environment set up to accommodate you? For example, if you're a light sleeper, are you stuck beside someone who is snoring, or on a busy street? Are you still letting your kids crawl into bed in the middle of the night? Do you get to wake up naturally or are you woken up by others or an alarm?

_____

_____

_____

_____

If you're in really bad condition now, what sent you over the edge? Shift work, family problem, health problem, work problem, PTSD?

_____
_____
_____
_____

What crutches do you rely on? Drugs, food, stimulants, obsessions? For how long?

_____
_____
_____
_____

How effective are they? How do you feel when you use them? Do you want to be free of them? Are you willing to do the work to be free of them?

_____
_____
_____
_____

Do any of your relatives have problems sleeping? For how long? What are their symptoms? Are they similar to yours? Do they have any tips you can try?

_____
_____
_____
_____

MEDITATIONS & VISUALIZATIONS

"Cleaning Pipes": A pipe full of white, cooling yet searing light suffuses your body and mind. Another pipe sucks anger, rage, shame, guilt, blame, regret, fear, worry and more from your mind and body. It is replaced with the white light and you feel yourself healing at the cellular level. Feel the white light move slowly around your body, and revel in its touch.

"Trash the Toxic Thought": Each time an angry or other toxic thought arises, see yourself placing it in a trash can, and replace it with something you are grateful for. Say to yourself, "this thought no longer serves me and I am replacing it with correct, helpful thinking."

"Exhale Toxic Thoughts": With each exhalation, feel a wave of toxic thoughts leaving your body. With each inhalation, breathe in the love, grace and joy that is yours when you open your mind and heart. You can also breathe in gratitude; with each inhalation, focus on something for which you are very grateful.

"Enjoy the Bed": Notice the sensation of the pillow under your neck, and the softness and comfort of the pyjamas/blankets all over your body. Feel the mattress support your heels, lower legs, upper legs, buttocks, back, shoulders and head, and notice how comfortable it is. Notice the quiet around you and send your antennae out into it.

Send Your Thoughts to Space: Notice your surroundings, then send your attention out your window, up into the night sky. Imagine the moon, and stars, and imagine yourself near them, touching them, free of the limitations of physicality. Visualize yourself leaving our atmosphere and casting your first gaze upon the flaming ball of our sun. Take your thoughts to the edge of our galaxy, and visualize a massive nebula, a star-birthing soup, in all of its glorious colors. Bring yourself back in to your bed, slowly, and notice how comfortable you are.

Breathing Meditation from Thich Nhat Hanh's <u>Peace is Every Step</u> (page 10).

> *Breathing in, I calm my body.* [inhale]
> *Breathing out, I smile.* [exhale]
> *Dwelling in the present moment* [inhale]
> *I know this is a wonderful moment.* [exhale][32]

"SIMPLIFY YOUR LIFE" CHECKLIST

- ☐ Reduce travel, long hours, and "wired" time.

- ☐ Cut out non-essential commitments. Don't spread yourself too thin. You can be an over-achiever again when your health problems are sorted out. Everyone will manage just fine without your giving 150%.

- ☐ Optimize your work time and tasks so that you can shorten your work day. Be a person who works smarter, not harder and longer.

- ☐ Don't be afraid to delegate and ask for help. Require more independence and self-reliance in children, and be willing to relinquish your control over every detail while you're under repair.

- ☐ Use commuting time and break time productively. Do some active meditations while driving, like sending kind thoughts to all the people that pass you and even to those who cut you off. This helps prevent road rage and keeps your mood light and bright. You can learn a language, listen to great tunes or audio-books, and interesting non-shock-jock news programs. Make it *you* time.

- ☐ Sneak in some extra exercise. If you can, get in some yoga or exercise during a break at work. A few minutes of stretching, a ten minute walk. If you work from home, give yourself permission to take short exercise breaks. The impact on your productivity and your back health is immediate.

- ☐ Commit to leaving your work at work, and not bringing it home with you. Turn off the phone and laptop if you can. Resist the temptation to check or answer your emails; they can wait.

- ☐ This goes for your head, too. Develop the discipline to be present in the moment and don't dwell on your work problems when you're not there. You can use a helpful mantra like "This is MY time. I focus it where I CHOOSE." You can say this to yourself when you find your thoughts straying back to work problems. As with any physical discipline, you have to practice doing this, and it gets easier with time and training.

- ☐ Set your boundaries gently and respectfully and stick to them. Others will follow your lead and do the same.

- ☐ Slow down a bit. Modern life has us in a constant rush. This approach to living makes us sick, mentally and physically, and there's no end to it unless you step back a bit. You don't need to move to a Tibetan monastery. Just take some reasonable measures. Remember to breathe deeply. Remember to be kind to strangers. Remember to talk less and listen more.

☐ Set limits about what happens at night, because you need peace and quiet. Don't sleep with your children. Don't sleep with your partner if he or she snores. Speak to everyone gently and respectfully about your needs and they will be grateful to help you.

☐ Cut out non-essential social activities and personal travel if it interferes with sleep training.

"WHAT CAN YOU DO TODAY TO HELP SOLVE YOUR PROBLEMS" CHECKLIST

☐ Book an appointment for counseling.

☐ Call a help line.

☐ Go to the library to take out some self help books and CDs, or watch the great gurus on YouTube.

☐ Join a grief or addiction support group.

☐ Come clean about your truth.

☐ Exercise four times per week.

☐ Pray.

☐ Acknowledge that you need something, like work-life balance.

☐ Ask for the help you need.

☐ Admit you made a mistake and ask for forgiveness.

☐ Accept that your house will not stay clean for more than ten minutes after you've cleaned it until your children are older.

☐ Declare an intention to be unbotherable by the judgments of others.

☐ Declare that you will stop comparing yourself to others.

☐ Set a family meeting or schedule an appointment with your boss or a colleague so you can state what is bothering you.

☐ Telephone a family member to explain why something he or she said or did made you feel deeply hurt.

☐ Write down a list of goals, actions and a timeline.

☐ Keep track of your progress and surround yourself with supportive listening materials.

☐ Create a vision board.

☐ Research your next career path for ten minutes each day.

☐ Find a community of like-minded people so you have someone to talk to.

☐ Meet with your spiritual guide or counselor.

ADJUST YOUR ENVIRONMENT FOR BETTER SLEEPING - CHECKLIST

This is a list of some environmental and habit changes you can consider to improve your sleep:

- [ ] Get off of drugs. Sleeping pills, marijuana, nicotine, caffeine, alcohol etc.
- [ ] Cut out processed foods, sugary foods, and genetically modified foods like corn and soy.
- [ ] Eat lightly so you don't burden your body trying to digest.
- [ ] Don't eat after supper.
- [ ] Prepare your own meals. Invest a bit of time and thought into streamlining this so it's not a burden.
- [ ] Have a regular bedtime, at the right time. Insomniacs should get to bed between 10-11pm.
- [ ] Keep the lights dim after 9pm.
- [ ] Don't watch TV for at least the hour before you go to bed.
- [ ] Don't watch angry television programs at night. While you're healing, fill your mind with more relaxing and helpful fare, rather than watching stressed-out people cope badly with their stress.
- [ ] Keep your bedroom, bed, and bedding tidy, clean, comfortable and light/ noise/interruption free. Gently banish your spouse and children if they are noisy and wake you up frequently.
- [ ] Ask for help to handle circumstances requiring frequent night-time interruptions, like caring for young children.
- [ ] Make sure your mattress and pillows are comfortable. If you wake up sore in the morning, but the soreness goes away during the day, this is your clue that you need to make a change.
- [ ] Establish a daily bedtime ritual that is relaxing and fun and doesn't involve electronics. Nice tea, a fun book, gentle stretching, meditation, a warm bath. Give yourself at least 3 weeks to train your body and brain to respond to the ritual; that's about how long it takes to make a habit stick.
- [ ] Don't turn on the television or your computer in the middle of the night. If you must get up, do some gentle stretching or read.
- [ ] Exercise daily, with harder exercise earlier in the day.

- ☐ Exercise outside, near water, forests, rivers etc.
- ☐ Try yoga and exercises where you need to more your arms around (this stimulates lymph drainage).
- ☐ Take a walk in the early morning sunlight to help set your clock.
- ☐ Figure out how to laugh more. Add this to your daily to-do list. Play with your children outside at night. Watch a funny video.
- ☐ Have more loving sex with your partner. Take the time for it, even if you feel like you don't have enough time. This is an investment that really pays off.
- ☐ Try some aromatherapy (like lavender)
- ☐ No family fighting at nighttime. Save serious talks for morning.
- ☐ Hold your tongue instead of lashing out at your family members when you're tired.
- ☐ Daily meditation and/or prayer, in the morning and evening.
- ☐ Do not obsess about your problems at night; you must change the mental channel. Instead, listen to helpful audio programs, books, music, and count your blessings.
- ☐ Shut off angry thoughts during the day, also, by focusing instead on gratitude and how you can bring positive change to your world.
- ☐ Practice patience with yourself and those around you.
- ☐ Take appropriate action during the day to handle the problems that bother you at night-time.
- ☐ Try some gadgets like an infrared sauna, grounding sheet, air filter, and magnetic therapy.

ABOUT THE AUTHOR

Rosanna D'Agnillo is a writer and musician living in Calgary, Canada with her husband and two sons. She experienced sleeping problems for many years, and severe insomnia for five years, before researching and writing this book so that she could share her drug-free healing journey. Please visit www.endinsomnia.com and www.rosannad.com for more books, articles, music and information.

Made in the USA
Charleston, SC
08 September 2013